7

A Carer's Odyssey

A Carer's Odyssey

Life as Mother, Wife, Carer

Anna Chan

Matador
5 Weir Road
Kibworth Beauchamp
Leicester LE8 0LQ, UK
Tel: 0116 279 2299
Fax: 0116 279 2277
Email: books@troubador.co.uk
Web: www.troubador.co.uk/matador

ISBN 978 1848765 733

British Library Cataloguing in Publication Data.
A catalogue record for this book is available from the British Library.

Typeset in 11pt Sabon by Troubador Publishing Ltd, Leicester, UK
Printed and bound in the UK by TJ International Ltd, Padstow, Cornwall

Matador is an imprint of Troubador Publishing Ltd

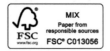

For Jeff and Emma

Contents

Acknowledgements

I am grateful to several Rett families and carers for allowing me to include their stories in the book. So many different stories, so many different kinds of courage, and so much inspiration.

Most of all I want to thank all the people who have helped and supported me in my role as a carer: friends, neighbours, family members, colleagues, the social, education and care professionals who work with my daughter Emma, the health professionals who support my husband Jeff and the charity workers who gave me advice and practical help. This has given the book a wide range and ensured an appeal to a wide audience.

Jeff deserves my special thanks for the wonderful parenting he supplies for Emma in spite of his own health problems and for cooperating with me in telling that story in Part 2.

Many thanks also to Brendan Hennessy for encouraging me to think about publishing and for his help at all stages.

Introduction

This book is about a journey – my journey of caring for my severely disabled daughter Emma and my husband Jeff who suffers from depression. It is also about the journey taken by other carers, and the knowledge and experience I have gained through my work as a Carers' Support Worker from April 2008 and my current work as Carers' Lead for an NHS Trust, from September 2009.

The odyssey has lasted, so far, for 18 years. It began when Emma was born, although for the first joyful year there was no hint of the pains, tribulations, trials and conquests to come. A child born with Rett Syndrome develops quite normally in the first year, then development starts to slow down. Skills that the child has acquired are lost. Rett Syndrome is a neurological disorder which causes severe physical and learning disability. The parents are faced with the challenge of getting to understand her and love her all over again.

Jeff and I were determined to do the best we could for Emma. We tried different therapies to improve Emma's mobility and communication. One of these included a trip to China with

Emma for cranial acupuncture treatment between November 1997 and February 1998. Although some of the therapies helped to improve Emma's abilities slightly, they were disruptive to our lives. In the end, Jeff and I decided it was more important to carry on with our lives as normally as we could.

We managed to do most things normal people do: work, school, holidays, etc. with the help of friends, family, neighbours and charitable organisations. Suddenly out of the blue, in January 2007 Jeff had a breakdown. This affected me badly both physically and mentally. I suddenly became two carers in one. We have moved to Part 2. I took voluntary redundancy from my work as a computer programmer at the end of 2007. So in a few months' time with the move into the caring profession, I was going to have three caring roles. And that takes us into Part 3.

This book is an update and expansion of an earlier self-published book *Getting to Know Emma,* which was based on a journal that I started in 1993. It was a way of coping with the burden. During Emma's early years, I had great difficulty in convincing the health and medical professionals that there was something wrong with her. The journal helped me to give detailed and accurate information to Emma's doctors and therapists. It also served as a confidant when I found that medical professionals, friends and family were not taking my concerns about Emma seriously. I spent many sleepless nights pouring my heart out to my willing, patient, non-judgemental and always available electronic friend – my personal computer.

Around 2001, I did a course in child development to help me to support Emma better. Most of the students were classroom assistants. At the end of the course, we had to do a talk about our experience of working with a child. I told the story of Emma and how I tried to help her to develop despite her disability and learning problems. I received such positive feedback from the lecturer and fellow students that I decided to write the story of Emma to help professionals to understand problems faced by parents of disabled children.

Turning the journal I kept into a book was much more difficult than I had anticipated. Old photographs, school and medical reports helped to refresh my memory, but producing a coherent account was difficult. I had not anticipated that writing the book would bring back the nightmarish memories. I often had tears streaming down my face onto the keyboard as I typed.

In 2002, with the help of Jeff, we managed to produce 200 copies of the book *Getting to Know Emma*. The book was handmade and we sold the book through friends and via a website. We had people buying the book from the USA, Canada and the Philippines – mainly from parents with disabled children and a few health and social care professionals.

Bringing the story up to date, I am inspired by the carers I meet and the remarkable progress made in finding a cure for Rett Syndrome as described in Appendix A. It was only after Jeff became ill that I realised I was a carer – one of the 6 million people in the UK caring for someone with a disability or illness. Since this book contains lengthy experience from both sides of caring – the professional as well as the personal – I hope it will be of benefit to both sides. I hope it will benefit anyone who has been confronted with similar burdens. I have aimed to convince the professionals and policy makers of the importance of working with families, of providing support for them.

My aim is even wider. I believe this book will encourage and inspire many other kinds of readers, both those who are confronting misfortunes of various kinds and those simply faced with daunting challenges. I have been inspired by numerous encounters, both in real life and discovered in the print and broadcast media. The unsung heroes described in Part 3 include some carers of exceptional humanity and dedication. Chapter 14 tells the stories of some of the severely disabled in various professions who have developed in compensation quite remarkable gifts not available to the 'normal'. In the Survival Guide and the Resources section can be found various kinds of help and support.

I would be interested to receive readers' comments on any aspects of the story. Please visit the website *www.acarersodyssey.com* to provide them and to get up to date.

Part 1

The Story of Emma

Chapter 1

A Late Developer

*The joys of parents are secret, and so are their
griefs and fears.*
Francis Bacon, Essays (1625)
'Of Parents and Children'

Jeff fell in love with Emma the moment he set eyes on her. She had thick dark hair and alluring chocolate brown eyes. She arrived on 6th December 1991, a week before the due date and she weighed 6lb 12oz. We were both elated. She was very precious to us; our first child. The midwife did an assessment on Emma's breathing, heart rate, skin colour, movements and response to stimulations one minute after she was born. After the assessment, she gave Emma an Apgar score of nine out of ten. The assessment was repeated five minutes after birth, and she scored ten out of ten. I was proud of her, my perfect baby. There was only one minor problem, Emma had a right 'clicking' hip. I was told that there was nothing to worry about. The joint usually grows back into the socket.

Emma was also very special for my family, the first grandchild for my parents and she was born on my sister Ann's 30th birthday. Jeff was so excited about Emma's arrival that he telephoned almost all the people in my address book. He phoned my colleagues at work, our friends, his family and my family, including my sister Mary in Australia.

My pregnancy had gone smoothly. I was fortunate that I did not experience any of the negative symptoms of pregnancy, no morning sickness or swollen ankles. The extra weight I put on during pregnancy had improved my normally anaemic and anorexic look. The hormone changes improved my skin considerably. I felt better than ever.

Emma's birth went well and I was proud that I did not need any pain relief. One problem was that I lost a lot of blood. I had to be taken to the ward from the delivery room in a wheelchair. They stopped the wheelchair outside the ward. Two nurses tried to help me to walk to my bed but I told them that I could manage. I managed the first and second steps. As I attempted the third step I collapsed and fainted. I was always too proud to receive help.

When I woke up a little later, Jeff was at my bedside holding Emma. She was wrapped in a beautiful white woollen shawl. Jeff handed Emma to me. It was wonderful holding her in my arms. I was so excited that I could not sleep that night.

The nurses at the hospital were helpful. During the five days in the hospital I learned a lot about looking after Emma. I made friends with other mothers on the ward, and we exchanged stories about our pregnancies and giving birth. I did feel slightly out of place being older than most other mothers. I was 32. The girl in the next bed was only 19. Her boyfriend had left her when he discovered she was pregnant. Fortunately, her mother was very supportive. I felt I was so lucky to have both Jeff and Emma.

I had great difficulty managing on my own after I came home from hospital. I was feeling tired and weak. Jeff had to go back to work and I was left alone with Emma. Both Jeff's mother and my mother lived too far away to provide practical help. My best friend Wai had delivered her first baby six weeks ago. Fortunately Christine, living opposite was most helpful. Her two sons Matthew, aged five, and Oliver, aged three, were fascinated by Emma. The visits from the midwife were a real godsend. One thing I learned from my fainting episode in the hospital was that I must not be too proud to accept help and I should be grateful to those who offer help.

We had many visitors after we came home: family, friends, colleagues and neighbours. The house was full of flowers and gifts. I was delighted that a baby could bring out such kindness from everyone.

We usually spend Christmas with Jeff's family in Warwick and then visit my family in Cheltenham afterwards, which involves a lot of travelling. That year we decided to spend Christmas at home. It was the first time we had done so. We bought a real Christmas tree and Jeff cooked the Christmas lunch. It was a magical time, I had never felt happier in my life.

I was not a natural mother. Emma's crying, her occasional skin problem and the sleepless nights upset me. I felt as helpless as a schoolgirl every time Emma cried or became sick. Babies are such illogical creatures. They have such a poor sense of timing, do not communicate clearly and are insensitive to other people's feelings. Worse still, I did not have any training in looking after babies.

Despite my inexperience as a mother, I made up for it in enthusiasm. I took her to the baby clinic every week, took her out for walks. I was amazed to see how good Jeff was with Emma. He was a natural. He was much more patient and calmer than I was. He helped to bathe and feed Emma, and he changed her nappies. Emma was his pride and joy. He loved taking her out in her pram to show her off to people.

It was early 1992. I took Emma out to the local park as often as I could. People would approach to look at her. They were all captivated by her angelic look. I always received a lot of complimentary comments about what a beautiful baby she was. Emma got her dark hair and dark eyes from me, the rest she inherited from Jeff.

Emma was a good baby on the whole. She fed well and slept well. She did all the things a normal baby did. She gurgled, moved her eyes when she heard a noise, moved her arms and kicked her legs. We were pleased with her progress in the first three months. She started sleeping through the night when she was two and half months. We noticed that she was very interested in music. My parents bought her a musical mobile which we hung over her cot. Every time we played the music to her, she would wave her hands and kick her legs enthusiastically.

The end of my maternity leave was fast approaching just when I was getting used to looking after Emma and staying at home. I had to admit that I was missing my work as a computer programmer and the company of my colleagues. I could have opted to take a two-year career break. There were three reasons for wanting to return. The first was the insecurity of Jeff's job. He escaped the first round of redundancies at the company where he worked and was transferred to the Head Office in the City but his post was only temporary. He was not sure whether he would find another IT post within the company after that. The second reason was my fear that my skills would become outdated in two years' time. The computing industry is highly competitive and the technology changes at frightening speed. The third reason was that the company that I worked for had taken over another company and my department urgently needed resources to carry out the transfer of data onto our own computer.

Once I had decided to return to work I was faced with the most daunting task every working mother has to face – finding a childminder. It was more difficult than I thought. I obtained a list of registered childminders from the council and phoned nearly everyone on the list. Either they did not have a vacancy or I found them not suitable. Two weeks before I was due back at work I still did not have a childminder. I was getting desperate.

I turned to my neighbour Christine for help. Originally, I had hoped that Christine could be Emma's childminder. Her second son Oliver had been ill and she had been spending quite a lot of time in the hospital with him. Anyhow, there was a possibility that the family would be emigrating to New Zealand because Christine's husband Ian had been offered a good job there. Fortunately, Christine was able to recommend Kate to us. Kate was the daughter of Christine's friend. She had been a nanny for nearly two years looking after a young baby of similar age to Emma.

Jeff and I went to see Kate. We were impressed with the cleanliness and the tidiness of her house. We had a chat with Kate and we were impressed with her knowledge and her experience with babies despite the fact that she was only nineteen. Kate was quiet, but she was sensible and practical. We decided that she was suitable.

Kate came round to babysit a few times before I went back to work so that she had a chance to get to know Emma, to find out her feeding pattern and the type of things Emma enjoyed. She got on well with Emma and I was confident that she would take good care of her.

The first day back to work in April was a traumatic experience. The night before I had got all the things ready, but when I got up in the morning I could not find anything I needed. I was in panic mode. I rushed around to get myself and Emma ready. Everything seemed to go wrong that morning. I found a hole in my tights, the cereal had run out and Jeff was in the bathroom for ages. To top it all, Emma was sick on my best cardigan just as I was about to leave the house with her.

I managed to sort things out and got to Kate's house with Emma. We were greeted by Kate's father, Michael, who was a very friendly man. I have never known anyone as cheerful as he first thing in the morning. Emma took to Michael straightaway. She gave Michael a big smile. I had a brief chat with Kate about Emma's feeding time and then I left for work.

I could not stop thinking about Emma all day long. A number of times I wanted to phone Kate to find out how Emma was getting on but I did not. It took a lot of self-control not to call. I thought she might be offended.

A number of things had changed since I left work six months ago. The procedure for logging into the computer system had been changed. It took me a few weeks to get back into the swing of things. Everyone in the office was interested in how Emma was doing and what she looked like. I had to describe her so many times that I put a photograph of her on my desk to show people what she looked like.

The first five weeks I worked part-time to ease my way back to work. After that I worked full-time. It was not too difficult once we worked out a system of delivering and collecting Emma. Kate was good with Emma and she seldom needed to phone me at work. Emma was also doing well. She started solid food when she was about four months old and she slept through the night most nights.

Emma continued to progress in the next few months and we were pleased with her. She sat up at five months and she could hold her bottle and feed herself at about six months. She started saying words like baa-baa, baby and boat. There was one particularly embarrassing word she kept saying – 'bugger'– and we did not know where she had picked it up from.

Emma was using her hands fairly well. She could hold a bread stick with her left hand and feed herself until she got to the end of it, then she would put it into her right hand and pick it up again with her left hand. She was also good with her pop-up zoo toy containing four buttons which required different actions to work. When the button was pressed or turned an animal would pop up. Emma managed three out of four buttons and she knew she had to close the lid to play again.

Both Jeff and I felt that we did not spend enough time with Emma in the evenings. We moved Emma's bedtime to about nine o'clock so that we could spend more time playing with her in the evenings. Some days I found it difficult to spend time with Emma after an exhausting day at work. We tried to make it up at weekends. We took Emma out to parks and playgrounds most weekends. She loved going on the swings.

When she was seven months old, we went to Coventry for

Jeff's niece Sharon's wedding. It was a church wedding and I was worried that Emma would misbehave during the ceremony. Fortunately she did not make too much noise. After the reception, we had a family gathering at Jeff's sister Carol's house. She made a lovely buffet dinner for us and Emma was fascinated by her cousin Steven's toys. Uncle Michael took some beautiful photographs of Emma that day. She was posing for him like a professional model. Steven brought down all his toys to show Emma. When Steven showed Emma his pet Syrian hamster, Emma said 'Doggie'. We were both amazed and amused by her. I remember that Emma's remark brought a lot of laughter.

My brother Kevin got married in September. My parents arranged for a big reception for over 200 people in a Chinese restaurant in Birmingham. My parents were very proud of Emma, taking her round, showing her off to our relatives. It was the first time some of my relatives had seen her. Everyone was won over by her angelic face and happy smile.

My friend Wai and I became closer because of our daughters. We lived about an hour's drive away from each other, but we kept in touch. We telephoned each other almost weekly to exchange news about the girls and met up as often as we could. Wai's daughter Cara was six weeks older than Emma but she was much more advanced. She had been walking by the age of ten months. I thought that this was due to the fact that Wai spent more time with Cara because she worked part-time. I told myself not to worry because children develop at different rates.

In October, we went to Cara's first birthday party. There were a few little girls and boys around the same age as Emma or slightly older. Most of them had started to walk. Emma was the only one who was not mobile; she had not even started to crawl. She just sat in the corner while the others rushed in and out of rooms. She was not interested in their toys. We tried to get Emma to join in, but she was not interested. She stayed rooted and staring at the same spot. When one boy accidentally burst a balloon, Emma screamed. From then on, the typical healthy one-year-old Emma that I had got to know began to be replaced by another Emma, equally loveable but a much greater challenge.

That was the first time I noticed that Emma was slower than the average child in several ways. When we got home, I telephoned my mother to find out what I was like when I was a baby. She told me that I was a lazy baby, I slept a lot and was not very active. I did not go through the crawling process, I just stood up and walked one day. I thought Emma was taking after me.

Around the same time, my neighbour Christine and her family emigrated to New Zealand, which was a great loss to me. I really missed their friendship and Christine's practical help and her down-to-earth opinions. I also missed her boys Matthew and Oliver coming around to see Emma and their incessant questions about everything.

We had a party for Emma's first birthday. She was in a bad mood that day and she did not take any interest in her presents or her cake. We were a little concerned about her anti-social behaviour. The others told us not to worry, Emma was just a little tired or she was not used to seeing so many people in the house.

Kate took Emma to see the health visitor for her first-year check up. I had wanted to take Emma myself, but I was too busy to take time off work. Everything was fine. Emma's weight and height were normal, her eyesight and hearing were fine. I was quite relieved to learn that everything was all right. Kate and I had quite a few discussions about how to motivate Emma to move and do things. We thought that stimulating toys might help. Emma already had quite a lot of toys from her first birthday. We went out and bought more toys but they did not help.

We took a long break at Christmas, about ten days off work. We spent Christmas with Jeff's parents and then we went to see my family. During the Christmas period, we tried everything we knew to encourage Emma to be more active but our efforts were in vain. We were disappointed at her lack of development. About two weeks after the New Year, we were pleasantly surprised that Emma had started to crawl – though more of a shuffle than a crawl.

It was 1993. Mobility gave Emma the opportunity to explore her surroundings and she did this with great enthusiasm. She pulled all the newspapers from the coffee table onto the floor and ripped them to shreds. She had a good time pulling off the leaves from the lower part of our weeping fig plant. She was everywhere and unstoppable. We had to move everything out of her reach. She enjoyed pulling Jeff's shoelaces off when he was sitting down. We had to warn our visitors to check their shoelaces before they left the house.

In February, my workload was less and I was able to take Emma to have her MMR injection. Emma cried a little when the nurse injected her but she was all right afterwards. She had a mild temperature in the afternoon, but it was a fairly normal reaction. I gave her some Calpol and her temperature was back to normal within a few hours. The following day Emma was fine.

From around March, Emma started to become very quiet. Every morning, when Michael opened the door to greet us, that wonderful smile had gone. We tried to teach Emma to wave goodbye, but she just stared into thin air. She had developed an interest in books, she would play incessantly with her books. She would turn the pages over until she reached the end, then she would start all over again.

In the evenings, we tried to play with Emma, but she would look away and carry on playing with her books. She became withdrawn and she would not look at people directly. Up to now, she had responded to her name quickly but now she would not turn her head. There was other odd behaviour. Emma lost interest in the swings. She was terrified of going on the slides. There was a blank look in her eyes when we tried out a new place or a new game with her.

In April, when Emma, aged one year and four months, developed a chest infection after a heavy cold, I took her to see our GP. I mentioned that I was worried that Emma was not developing normally like other children. My GP told me not to worry: children develop at different rates, Emma was just a little slow and she would catch up in a few months' time. Unfortunately, this was not the case. We discovered more problems during our two-week holiday in Hong Kong.

Chapter 2

What's Wrong with Emma?

Children sweeten labours, but they make
misfortunes more bitter.
Francis Bacon, Essays (1625)
'Of Parents and Children'

Our holiday in the summer of 1993 in Hong Kong was to be a special holiday, the first visit for Jeff. I had wanted to show Jeff around Hong Kong for years. It was more than just a holiday for me, it was an opportunity to visit the place of my birth. It also gave me a chance to see my brother, John, my relatives and friends. My sister Mary and her fiancé Geoff would be joining us in Hong Kong from Australia. It was to be an exciting holiday with lots of places to visit, people to see and food to taste.

Behind all the excitement I was a little worried about travelling such a long distance with Emma. It was the first time I had travelled on a plane with her and the packing was a mammoth task; deciding on what to take and what to leave at home was a real headache. I made the mistake of not packing spare clothes in the hand luggage.

Emma was well behaved at the airport and during the first half of the flight. Then she started to get bored and became restless. The air hostess tried to play with Emma, but she was not interested. She wanted to eat everything we were given. We just gave her everything she wanted to pacify her so that she did not disturb other passengers. Later Emma was sick, she vomited all over her own clothes and my trousers. I took her to the toilet to wash her and myself. But the stains and the smell could not be washed away. The rest of the journey was uncomfortable, to say the least.

Mary and Geoff were looking forward to seeing Emma. They were captivated by her angelic looks, but they were disappointed at her attitude. She was totally uninterested in them and would not look at them. She reacted in the same way to my friends, relatives and other people who came to see her. Emma's Eurasian features (English features from Jeff and Chinese features from me) attracted a lot of attention wherever we went. People would come up to her and pinch her cheek and say: 'Hello, pretty girl' – a typical Chinese way of showing fondness to children. Emma would just ignore them by turning away or give them a blank look. I felt embarrassed about her behaviour and I just told people that she did not understand Cantonese. However, I knew that was not the reason.

We saw many children while in Hong Kong. Chinese people took their children with them everywhere, even to restaurants. I noticed that children younger than Emma could do more. They could point at things, wave goodbye, hold food in their hands and feed themselves, and run around. Emma could not do any of these things and I could not understand why. I was getting worried. Even the excitement of Hong Kong failed to distract me from these worries.

On the whole, our holiday was enjoyable. Emma was the only person who did not seem to enjoy it. It was hot and she slept a lot. She was sick a number of times, once at a reunion with my university friends and once at a department store. At the time, I thought it was caused by the herbs and spices in Chinese food which Emma was not used to eating.

I was often asked why Emma was not talking or walking. I just did not know how to answer. A number of people suggested that it was the childminder not spending enough time teaching her to do things. They told me horror stories about some Filipino maids who gave their babies sedatives or alcohol so that they could go out and see friends. I had doubts about the truth of these stories but I could not help thinking that perhaps Kate was not doing the right things with Emma.

I had been thinking about taking Emma to a day nursery or to another childminder with more children. The first option was not feasible because all nurseries in the borough only took children between the ages of two and five. Emma seemed to be happy at Kate's even though she was not progressing, so I decided to leave Emma with Kate until she became two years old in December.

As there was not much I could do to change Emma's day care,

I thought I would find out what I could do at home with Emma to help her to develop. I contacted the health visitor and asked her to visit. Our usual health visitor was off sick and another one came in her place. As she did not know Emma, I gave her an account of Emma's developmental history. I asked her whether she thought Emma might have some physical problems which affected her movements. She checked Emma's health record and everything was normal. The health visitor told me that it was nothing to worry about and that Emma was just a late developer. Then she asked me whether I worked full time and whether I had tried to teach Emma Chinese as well as English. She seemed to think that my working full time might be affecting Emma's development. She said that Emma might get confused if I taught her to speak two languages which was not the case. I was deeply upset by her questions even though I knew she was only trying to be helpful.

After observing Emma for a while, the health visitor told me that there was nothing wrong with Emma physically. She just needed motivation to encourage her to move and to do things. She suggested that we should motivate Emma to move by putting her bottle or her favourite toy out of her reach. She demonstrated this by putting Emma's bottle on her chair, but Emma did not show any interest in it. The health visitor then sang 'Round and Round the Garden' and Emma listened with great interest, which was unusual. She sang a few other songs, and Emma smiled. I was pleased that Emma was responding.

We tried out the singing method on Emma and it was

successful. Emma's eye contact improved when we sang to her. I was amazed at how well she could remember the songs. When I sang 'Round and Round the Garden' to her, she would start giggling just when I reached the part 'One step, two step and tickle under there'. We also tried the 'Putting Objects Out-of-Reach' trick but the success rate was variable, depending on the object we used and the mood Emma was in. We managed to get Emma to pull herself up from the ground onto the sofa and to climb a few steps up the stairs.

We bought some cassette tapes and videos. She loved them. She could concentrate for a long time while watching the videos and she would gently rock herself when her favourite songs came on. She also started pulling herself up and moved around, holding onto the sofa and other furniture. We were pleased with her progress. We tried to get her to walk without support, but she was too frightened to let go.

While I was pleased with the small progress Emma was making with music and mobility, I was a little disturbed by the two irritating habits she had acquired; curling her toes and sucking her fingers. Emma curled her toes inwards when she was sitting down. If I tried to straighten them out she would curl them up again. She also started putting her hand in her mouth a lot. I first noticed Emma sucking her fingers when I was at my work manager's barbecue in August. I remember that I tried to stop her several times but she would not stop. My colleagues told me not to worry, it was natural for children to do that.

I was rather puzzled by her new habits. I did not understand why Emma, who had never sucked her fingers or a dummy before, would suddenly start sucking her fingers. Thinking it must be boredom, I discussed it with Kate and we agreed that Emma should go to a playgroup to play with other children. Looking back at our holiday photographs a few months later, I discovered that Emma had started her bad habits much earlier than I had thought. The photographs we took in June showed that Emma was already sucking her fingers and curling her toes.

Since our holiday in Hong Kong, Jeff's mind was preoccupied with the threat of redundancy. He knew that he did not stand a good chance because he was new to the department and the area in which he was working was targeted for cuts. I knew he had not been happy at work and we worked out that we could manage for a few years on his redundancy money and my salary. With this reassurance, Jeff decided to apply for Voluntary Separation.

Meanwhile, I was keeping a close observation on Emma. I noticed sometimes when I woke her up in the morning that she breathed in an odd manner. She breathed in deeply and then held her breath for a short while. I also noticed that when Emma was sitting down playing or watching television, occasionally she would open her hands outward, throw her head backward and roll her eyes back in such a way that only the whites were visible. I told Jeff about this, but he told me not to worry about it, Emma was just playing about. I was rather annoyed by Jeff's attitude. I had also mentioned

Emma's strange behaviour to friends, but they did not seem to think it was anything to worry about. I became more and more worried about Emma's inexplicable behaviour.

One Sunday afternoon in September, we took Emma to our local park. We put her on the swing and Emma was all right for a few minutes and after that she lost interest and looked frightened, so we took her off. We tried the slide and Emma was terrified. So Jeff decided to get Emma to walk. I sat down on a bench and watched them. It was quite a comical sight, a six-foot tall man walking with this tiny girl.

While I was watching them, a woman came and sat next to me. She started the conversation first by asking about Emma's pushchair. Later our conversation became focussed on Emma. This woman was friendly and understanding, and I felt at ease talking to her. Sometimes it is easier to confide your worries to strangers.

Her name was Lesley. I told her about Emma's development history, my worries and the lack of support from the medical profession and the scepticism from my friends and family. After listening to my story and watching Emma play for a while, Lesley said: 'From what you have told me, and watching Emma's movements, I think there's something wrong with her. You really ought to take her to your GP and get her to refer Emma to a paediatrician'. Her remarks startled me. It was not the usual comforting words that I was used to hearing. I later discovered that Lesley had been a paediatric nurse for over 20 years.

I took Emma to see my GP and told her that I was concerned about Emma not talking or walking. I was adamant that tests should be carried out. The GP saw the way Emma was walking and thought there might be something wrong with her legs and arranged for Emma to have them X-rayed at a local hospital. Also she referred Emma to a paediatrician based at a pre-school assessment centre.

Jeff's application for Voluntary Separation was approved and he left the company on 17th October. About the same time, Emma started walking independently. She just pulled herself up on a chair, took her hands off the chair and walked to the sofa opposite. We could not believe our eyes. It was a great joy for us to see her walking. However, I still believed that there was something not right about her and I wanted to know what.

In November, we found a place at a local nursery for Emma to attend in January 1994. I expected it to be a difficult transition from being with Kate to being at a nursery. Jeff decided to help Emma to ease into her new environment by taking her to the nursery for a few hours a week. This worked well, Emma fitted in well.

It was also a big transition for Jeff. He found himself working from home and self-employed after doing a nine-to-five office job for over 20 years. I was worried about Jeff running a business: he was good working with computers, but not with marketing or communicating with people. Jeff's computer consultancy business was not a success, but that turned out to be a blessing in a way. In the months to follow, he was able to spend a lot more time with Emma when she needed him the most – as her condition was worsening. It was wonderful that he made such a quick bond with Emma. He also gave me the support I needed to carry on working and the strength I needed to keep my sanity.

I thought that once I had got over the hurdle of getting my GP to refer Emma, the rest would be easy. I naïvely believed that it would not be long before we found out the cause of Emma's development problems. The X-ray taken in September was the first in a series of tests and assessments that Emma underwent. The X-ray photographs on Emma's legs did not reveal anything wrong with her bones. They looked normal.

About two months later, on the 10th November we saw a speech and language therapist to have Emma assessed. The report said that Emma had speech and language problems and advised that Emma would benefit from speech therapy. In December, Emma went to see the senior educational psychologist and she advised taking Emma to a local development assessment centre for children with special needs.

I went to see the head of the assessment centre in December, and saw what they did for the children. Emma, now two, was admitted on 14th January 1994. Later we saw the paediatrician at the centre and we had about an hour's session with her. At the first session it was just a simple test with Emma to see if she could pick things up; big things and small things. The physiotherapist was there at the same time. They were observing what Emma could do and we discovered that she could do very little. She could not do any of the things they asked her to do. The paediatrician organised a series of tests in February. The results were normal except for the blood test. The result revealed a high level of German Measles antibodies in Emma's blood. She explained that it could be caused by me catching German Measles during pregnancy or Emma catching it after she was born. I found it hard to believe that I had failed to notice either Emma or myself having German Measles. However, the thought that some illness of mine could have caused Emma's problem made me sick with guilt.

I went to the library near work to look this up. After consulting a number of medical journals, I realised that Emma's condition could not have been caused by German Measles damage when she was inside me. Because if I did have German Measles while I was pregnant, Emma's problems would have been apparent at birth. Her lungs and other organs would have been badly damaged as well as her brain. But Emma's development was normal in her first year.

The paediatrician decided that Emma should continue with hearing and eyesight tests, and later a brain scan and an Electroencephalograph (EEG). The tests revealed nothing abnormal. I decided to start keeping an account of Emma's development so far. I put in it things that I had not told other people before – Emma could say words like 'Baby, Baba, Boy,

Dada, Mumma and Doggie' when she was seven months old, and that she was able to play with toys like the Pop-Up Zoo but that these skills had disappeared. I had not mentioned my observations to the medical profession before because of the difficulty in convincing them that Emma was not developing normally. I feared that if I mentioned this loss of skills they would think that I was making it up or imagining it. But children do not lose skills as they grow for no apparent reason. I submitted the report to the paediatrician and hoped that it would help.

At this point, Emma was attending the local nursery for four days a week and the assessment centre one day a week. We had hoped that the stimulation Emma received from being with other children at the nursery and the special education at the centre would boost her development, but there was no improvement. In fact, Emma's behaviour had continued to deteriorate since January. She had started to grind her teeth and wring her hands, and had been sucking her hands more often. She sucked her hands so much that the skin became split and looked very sore. We tried putting foul tasting things on her hands but she was not deterred.

Even though Emma had been able to walk independently since the previous October, we had only managed to get her to walk outdoors from February. She had this peculiar way of stopping whenever she came across something that was a different colour or texture. It took us a few weeks to persuade her to walk on grass.

The worst problem was Emma's crying. She would cry for no apparent reason. Sometimes a crying session would last for over three hours. We tried everything to console her but failed miserably. Her crying drove both Jeff and I to distraction. Emma's incessant crying also upset our neighbours. They came over once to ask why Emma was crying so much and all we could say was that we did not know, that we wished we knew how to stop her. They must have thought that we were neglecting Emma or ill-treating her. Occasionally, they got so frustrated by the noise that they banged on the wall, which upset me immensely.

Eventually, we found two activities that helped. Walks had a calming effect on her and so did videos of songs and nursery rhymes. Music videos were most effective. She became so mesmerised by the music that she would stop sucking her hands or grinding her teeth.

There were further tests. She had an appointment with the neurologist on 12th May and then on 7th July she had a brain scan at a local hospital. The latter was a traumatic experience, both for us and for Emma. We took her to the hospital at 10am and she was not allowed to have anything to eat or drink for four hours previously. They gave her a general anaesthetic before the scan. She did not wake up until about 7:30pm.

I became more and more obsessive about Emma's condition. I started reading medical dictionaries. I had read a lot about childhood illnesses but nothing seemed to match Emma's condition. The closest I found was autism. Emma displayed some of the classical symptoms, lack of interest in her surroundings and avoiding eye contact. I contacted the National Autistic Association and was told a test could not be done until Emma was at least three years of age. I started to collect articles from newspapers and magazines. I kept talking to friends and colleagues about Emma's condition, I kept going over her reports, reading medical articles, analysing her development.

Emma had an EEG test on 27th July. This was not as bad as I had expected. We took her to the hospital in the afternoon. The test didn't take long. It involved putting a lot of electrodes on Emma's head and measuring the brain waves being emitted. This she did under normal conditions and she had another test under flashlight activity, because under flashlights her brain should respond much more, and the whole thing took about half an hour. We left the hospital thinking that the result would be like all the other tests – no conclusion. We knew that Emma's brain scan was normal and thought that her EEG would be too.

Whenever I talked about Emma to other people I got quite different reactions. Some people dismissed me as being neurotically over-anxious. Some people, because I am a working mother, thought that I had neglected Emma, and that was why she developed so slowly. Others were sympathetic, they encouraged me to do more to get Emma's condition diagnosed. Most people said 'Oh, don't worry. Emma will grow out of it'. They would quote examples of children they knew who were also late developers in some way. They would say 'So-and-so didn't speak until he was three years old' or 'So-and-so didn't walk until she was nearly four'. Some would give examples of famous people like the Victorian historian Macaulay who was silent until the age of six when he suddenly began lecturing his parents.

Emma's problem affected me both physically and emotionally. The constant worry gave me sleepless nights causing me to lose weight. My weight went from seven and a half stones down to under seven stones. Jeff used to joke that I was so weak that I could not even be a Seven-Stone Weakling! I developed back pain and a wrist strain as a result of carrying and lifting Emma. Emotionally I became very fragile. I cried a lot during my sleepless nights. I became impatient with Emma. I also became angry with people not believing that Emma had a development problem. Sometimes I felt I was losing my ability to cope and would have a breakdown.

Jeff had been supportive during those difficult months. He delivered and collected Emma to and from the nursery and the centre. He looked after her at home when she went down with infections, which happened quite frequently in the winter months. He took Emma to undergo tests. He also took her walking every day, which we later discovered was vital to retaining Emma's mobility. However, Emma's condition placed an enormous strain on our relationship. Sometimes when I looked back, I thought I was fortunate to get through this trauma without a nervous breakdown or marriage breakup.

I looked back at Emma's appointments and reports to try to figure out what was wrong with her. Her condition was puzzling not only me but also the medical and health professionals who worked with her. Appendix B shows a list of the tests and assessments Emma underwent. I went through this list over and over again. I thought to myself that if all these tests did not show anything perhaps there was nothing wrong with Emma after all. What was the point of all these tests? I had to sit and watch needles being inserted into Emma again and again, seeing her being wired up so many times, all without any answers.

Emma had to undergo more hearing and sight tests in August and a neurology test in September. Then we received another letter asking us to bring Emma to take another EEG test on the 13th September. The first EEG must have shown something wrong.

Chapter 3

A Shocking Diagnosis

Deep, unspeakable suffering may well be called a baptism, a regeneration, the initiation into a new state.
George Eliot

The answer came on Thursday, 8th September 1994, a day that I would never forget. I went to work as usual that morning and I had a very busy day at work and did not arrive home until nearly 7pm. I opened the front door and shouted: 'I'm home. How's Daddy and Baby?' There was no answer. I went to the living-room and saw Jeff sitting on the sofa and Emma sitting on the floor watching her favourite video, *The Makaton Nursery Rhyme*. I asked Jeff how the neurology test went and he did not answer. Then I saw this terrible pained expression on his face and I knew something awful had happened.

I went up to him and asked him what was wrong. It took him a while to come out with the words 'Emma has Rett Syndrome'. He was in tears as he spoke. I had not seen Jeff cry before and it shocked me. I asked the inevitable question:

'What is Rett Syndrome?' Jeff gave me a photocopy of an extract from a medical dictionary which he had found in the local library. My hands shook in disbelief as I read it.

Rett Syndrome is a multi-handicapping neurological disorder. It occurs approximately one in 10,000 female births. It is thought to be caused by the mutation of a gene of the X-chromosome. Characteristics include loss of skills after an early period of seemingly normal development, regression in social development, severe learning difficulties, development of repetitive hand movements, hyperventilation, grinding of teeth, curvature of spine and seizures. There is no known cure for Rett Syndrome. Drugs can be used to control seizures. Physiotherapy and hydrotherapy are useful in improving muscle tone. Unfortunately, an independent life is never possible for sufferers.

The symptoms matched Emma's condition but the prognosis was so bleak. I cried hysterically while Jeff tried to console me. Emma was oblivious of what had happened, she was so mesmerised by the music. I looked at Emma, so sweet, so innocent and so beautiful. How could something so cruel and horrific happen to her? With no cure available, Emma would be totally mentally and physically disabled for the rest of her life. We had been in the dark for so long, not knowing what was wrong with Emma and why she was behaving in such strange ways. Now, it all became clear and we felt powerless.

After I had calmed down, I managed to get the details of the appointment from Jeff. Emma had been to the nursery as usual in the morning. Jeff went to pick her up at about 11:45am to get to the assessment centre just after noon. He and Emma were called to see a senior neurologist from a London hospital, about a quarter of an hour later. He expected to see just the neurologist there, but there was also the paediatrician, the physiotherapist and two other medical staff. He thought that something must be up. The neurologist asked a few questions about Emma, how she was getting on, how she was walking and so on. The neurologist observed Emma for a while, noting the repetitive hand movements and the awkward, jerky movements. She asked Jeff if Emma would walk across the room. Jeff got up and made Emma walk towards the neurologist by pushing her. After watching Emma walk, the neurologist told Jeff that she thought Emma had Rett Syndrome. Jeff had never heard of it before.

The neurologist said that she was almost certain that was what Emma had, but would want to confirm it with another specialist in about two months' time. She also said that Emma would have difficulty walking and talking and said that she would require special educational needs. Jeff said that she was already going to the centre class two and a half days a week and went to a normal day nursery for the other two and a half days a week. The neurologist went on to say that girls with RS live to be adults in their forties. She said that Emma's health and educational needs would be carefully monitored and said that the centre would refer us to the Rett Syndrome Association UK (RSAUK).

After Jeff had finished, I told him that I did not want to go to work the following day. I could not face seeing people and I did not want people to see me in such a pitiful state. But Jeff said: 'We must carry on our lives as normal. We must be strong for Emma'. He was right, we had to be strong – both physically and mentally. We needed to make plans for the future, we needed to do our best for Emma. We sat down to discuss what we needed to do next. Should we tell people of Emma's disorder ; if so who would we tell and how much would we tell?

It was a coincidence that my friend Grace phoned that evening to see whether she could come over to have a shower because John was re-tiling the bathroom. I broke down in tears as I spoke to her, and she said she and John would come over to see us. Grace and John were good friends of ours. We had met them at a Chinese Association function a few months before and we became close friends quickly because Grace and I had a lot in common.

Grace and John arrived about half an hour later. They taught at special schools and they had not heard of RS before. They were sympathetic. They must have seen many parents with special needs children. They stayed and talked with us for nearly two hours. It was comforting to know that we had such caring and supportive friends.

We asked for their advice on whether we should tell the teachers at the nursery and our parents. They advised us not to tell our parents until we had all the facts. As for the nursery, we were not under any obligation to tell them. We should tell them when we were ready to do so. We also asked for their advice on special schools and other things. They gave us a lot of information. Before they left, John promised to look up RS at his school library which specialised in books on all kinds of disabilities.

That night, I had great difficulty getting to sleep. I lay in bed tossing and turning, trying to take in this terrible news. I tried to make sense of why this had happened to Emma. Was it something inherited from Jeff or me, or was it an accident of nature?

According to the medical dictionary, one in 10,000 girls is affected by this disorder. I have never had any luck with lotteries. I have never won anything in raffles or prize draws. Why had this rare disorder struck my daughter? My grief gave way to anger. I wanted to know why this had happened to me.

I did not smoke or drink and I had done all the right things during my pregnancy. I took vitamin tablets, did as much exercise as I could and gave up eating all the things that I was not supposed to eat during pregnancy. I had been faultless and yet my daughter had been born with this profound handicap. Some women smoked, drank or took drugs while pregnant and yet they had normal and healthy babies. Why was life so unfair?

Was it a punishment for something I had done? It is a common Chinese belief that children received punishments for the wrongdoings of their parents. I had never done anything to harm anyone; I had not stolen, robbed, cheated or committed murder. Why had this happened to me? It did not make sense.

Three o'clock, I decided that I needed sedatives to help me to sleep. I tried not to become dependent on them, but in the next few months I seldom managed to get to sleep without them. I woke up the next morning feeling drowsy and when I looked into the mirror I had a shock seeing the state I was in. I forced some breakfast down and drove off to work. Half way to work I realised my car was almost out of petrol, My mind was so preoccupied with Emma, I could not think about anything else.

On the following Monday, Yvonne Milne, the chairperson of the RSAUK, telephoned. She told Jeff not to be too worried about what he had read in the medical journals because they often describe the worst-case scenario.

An information pack arrived on Saturday morning. I took it upstairs and we read it in bed. It was very informative and helpful. As I read one article which said that all the Rett girls have pretty faces and alert eyes, and their eyes show such mystery and sadness. I could not help bursting into tears. Such irony! Such tragedy! I showed it to Jeff and he cried too for those beautiful lost girls.

On Sunday 18th September, I started typing out the journal. It took me about three hours to type up the events since

Emma's diagnosis. In the afternoon we took Emma out for a long walk in a local park. Emma's walking had deteriorated since the summer holidays because she did not have to walk to the assessment centre any more. It was quite difficult walking with her because you had to drag her most of the time, and she tumbled a few times. After a while my wrists started hurting because of the effort of pulling her along. I became quite conscious that people were giving her strange looks because of the way she walked and constant sucking of her hands. Jeff was very good with Emma and we managed to walk her for about an hour non-stop, which was quite an achievement for her.

When we got home I asked Jeff, 'Can we put up with people giving Emma strange looks because of the way she walks and acts?' Jeff said, ' I suppose we will have to.'

Later in the afternoon I telephoned my mother. She had just visited my grandmother in Newcastle. She told me that she and my father would be going back to Hong Kong around the end of October for a long holiday. I asked her if she would come and stay with us for a few days before she went. She said that she was too busy with her work in the takeaway. I nearly told her that Emma had RS and that her condition might worsen, but I decided to hold back. She said that she was pleased that Emma was making progress and she thought that Emma would start talking once she turned three years old.

I woke up early again on Monday morning. I was surprised

that I did not cry. Perhaps typing out the diary had released my anger and emotions. Perhaps my tear ducts had dried up and I could not produce any more tears. I lay in bed and thought about what to tell my parents about Emma. After thinking hard I decided not to tell them the truth until they returned to England the following February. They had worked hard all their lives and they were so looking forward to their retirement. I could not spoil it for them. Besides, there was nothing they could do to help while they were in Hong Kong. I also decided not to tell Jeff's parents the whole truth about Emma. They were old and frail; I did not think that they could take the news.

But I did start to inform other members of my family, starting with my sister, Mary. On Sunday 9th October I telephoned her in Melbourne, Australia. She said that she had never heard of RS before, which did not surprise me, even though she was a nurse. She accepted the news calmly, as I had expected. She had suspected that there was something wrong with Emma during our holiday together in Hong Kong in July the previous year. I told her a little about the illness and gave her the address of the Australian Rett Syndrome Association. She said that she would contact the association and find out more about the illness. I also asked her to look up some information about a new drug used in the treatment of RS. Mary told me it should be no problem as she was studying at Victoria University and she had access to the medical library and the computer database.

In the following two weeks, I managed to inform my two

brothers and three sisters. They all agreed that we should keep the news from our parents until after they had their long holiday in Hong Kong.

We attended the 10th RSAUK annual conference at the Forte Hotel in Coventry between the 14th and 16th October. I had mixed feelings about the conference. There were two reasons why I wanted to attend. The first was to see Dr. Alison Kerr who is the advisor on RS, so that Emma could get a definite diagnosis. The second was to learn as much as possible about RS from other families and the professionals so that we could do our best for Emma. They were good reasons for attending but I was not certain whether I could cope with meeting the older RS girls and women, with seeing what advanced stages of the disorder were like.

The conference was spread out over two and half days, starting Friday afternoon and ending Sunday afternoon. Friday afternoon was for meeting other families. We talked with them and shared experiences. It was good to be able to talk to people who understood. It was strange to see the girls together. They suffered from the same condition, but their symptoms were quite different; they had their own ways of wringing and clapping their hands.

Saturday was more formal; talks and workshops run by the professionals. The conference was well organised. There were childminders to look after the girls while the parents attended the meetings and workshops. There was a team of American scientists from Oregon to give talks on the research developments and practical advice on helping the children.

There were families from Bulgaria, Hungary and Iceland. A team of doctors from Nottingham was there to carry out tests on breathing and swallowing. We took Emma for the tests and her breathing and swallowing were fine. We also attended two workshops. The first one was on physiotherapy – we learned some useful tips on massaging the feet to improve circulation and how to lift a child out of bed. The second workshop was on music therapy – we learned how to encourage the child to take part in music making.

The hotel foyer was full of displays of special toys and equipment for helping the girls to develop. There were books and videos on RS for sale. There were information displays on claims and benefits for the girls and their families. There were also cards and T-shirts for sale to raise money for the RSAUK.

Everyone was friendly and I felt a special bond with the people there. The disabilities of our daughters gave us a common purpose in life. One of the families I met was the Ravenscroft family. Heidi was round 30 at the time. Her parents Anne and Reg were devoted to her. Anne's dedication was recognised when she won the Daily Mail Carer of the Year award in May 2010. Her story is among those of other unsung heroes in chapter 13.

I had to admit that I was upset when I saw the older girls walking in tiptoes, and women in wheelchairs and with curved backs. I kept telling myself that things would be different when Emma started to grow into adulthood. On the whole, I was quite successful in controlling my emotions. There was just one occasion when I failed to control my tears – during the interval between talks, there was a slide show of the photographs of Rett girls sent in by parents. There was music playing in the background. The pictures of the girls and the words from Johnny Mathis's song *When a Child is Born* were too much for me to bear. Tears came rolling down my cheeks.

On Sunday we saw Dr. Kerr and she gave Emma a definite diagnosis of RS. Later on she gave a talk on her research. The talk was illuminating and also gave us a lot of hope that a cure was possible. We came away from the conference feeling more positive because we knew that there were people out there who understood and could give us help and support. It was also reassuring to know that scientists all over the world were doing research to find a cure and to improve the diagnosis rate. We knew it that it would take some time, but at least the work had been started.

We stayed with Jeff's parents in Warwick during the weekend of the conference. We told them that Emma had been diagnosed as suffering from a nervous disorder and that she would have difficulty in learning and doing things for herself. We did not think that it was appropriate to tell them about the severity of the disorder. Jeff's brother and his family came to visit on Saturday evening. We told them about Emma's diagnosis and gave them an information leaflet.

A few weeks after the conference, we decided to tell the teachers at the nursery about Emma's disorder. I had been terribly worried that they would say that they could not cope with Emma and we would have to take her somewhere else. Fortunately, they were very good about it and told us that they were managing all right with Emma. Besides, Emma was happy there, and the children and the teachers got on well with her.

There were so many uncertainties in this new role of being parents of a severely disabled child. We were not certain whether we would be able to meet this challenge. We needed more than just sympathy and understanding, we needed to find closer ties with people to share our experience and people who could give us guidance. We needed a more suitable place to bring Emma up in – a new environment would give us greater confidence.

We found that new environment in January 1995 when we moved house. After Emma's diagnosis, I had been determined to move to a bigger, detached house. Emma's constant crying continued to make our relationship with our next door neighbour difficult. With the diagnosis, it was apparent that Emma's crying was not a temporary problem. I knew that moving house was the only thing that would settle my mind. I wanted no more worry about upsetting the neighbours. Anyway, Emma would be happier in a bigger house with more space to move about.

We put our house on the market and started looking for a

suitable property. We used an estate agency that was a subsidiary of the bank I worked for. They found us a buyer within two weeks. Jeff found a house in the next town about six miles away. It did not look promising from the photograph but Jeff insisted I should take a look. When we walked into the house for the first time, I could see a smile on Emma's face. She felt so at home with the place and she walked around without hesitation. The house was chalet style built in the early 1970s. It had an L-shaped open plan lounge and dining room. It was light and airy. We liked the house straight away.

The house met most of our requirements. Jeff and I discussed it when we got home and we decided to put in an offer. It was totally uncharacteristic of us to make such a hasty decision. Whatever we had done in the past, we had planned months in advance, considering the pros and cons and making contingency plans. The new house was wonderful for Emma. She had more space to move around and she did not have to worry about bumping into furniture. It was wonderful for us. We did not have to worry about our neighbours and the assessment centre was still nearby.

We settled in quickly. Jeff made friends with the neighbours on either side. A few weeks after we moved in, a hand-delivered letter landed on our doormat. It was a letter from our neighbour from behind who offered to sell land to extend the rather small garden. Jeff went to see them, a couple called Tony and Joan. They had a 180ft long garden. Tony was in a wheelchair and he did not want the responsibility of looking after a large garden. We decided to buy the land from them. Jeff went to see Tony and Joan about the details during the process of selling. Not long after we bought the land, Jeff and Emma saw Joan in the local shopping area, and Joan told Jeff that Tony had died. I bought a card and asked Jeff to take it to Joan.

Once we had settled in, Jeff started applying for jobs because we had taken on a large mortgage. In May, Jeff found a temporary job manning the computer information help desk and he had to start in two days time. We could not find anyone to look after Emma for the time between her coming home after the assessment centre and us returning from work. After considering all sorts of possibilities, I thought of Joan.

I had to walk through the back garden consisting of 100 ft of densely grown bramble and stinging nettles to get to Joan's back door. She was sitting in her kitchen. I knocked on her door and it startled her as she did not expect to see anyone at her back door. Joan opened the door and I introduced myself. I explained to her that we needed someone to help to look after Emma after school. She had met Emma before and knew that she was disabled. She agreed to help. It was the beginning of a great friendship. She did not just help to look after Emma, she was a source of comfort to Jeff and me. Her experience of her husband's disability made her an ideal support. Joan is a good listener, always gives good advice. She is a treasure.

We also found comfort and support from the local Rett network. We got in touch with a Rett family nearby in

October 1994. Through this family, we joined a group of RS families near where we live. In our get-togethers, we exchange information about schools, medicines, support facilities and share our worries and frustrations. We have been together for a few years now, and we are like an extended family. This is all described in chapter 4.

Our local Mencap charity was a great help to us. We made good use of their library which had specialised books and toys for disabled children. Their child-minding service is efficient. They found Emma an excellent child-minder Jacque to look after her. They also organised special events such as a Christmas party and days out in the summer.

Getting Emma a place in a local school was also a big help. As Emma was getting older, the nursery found it increasingly difficult to meet Emma's needs. She needed a place that would be a logical upgrade from the nursery and the assessment centre. We asked the local authority to find Emma a suitable place and she started attending a special unit within a mainstream school full time in June 1995. Her teacher Elaine was a breath of fresh air, very positive and enthusiastic. She brought Emma out of her shell, she was happier and more responsive. We had been sceptical about whether Emma was capable of learning and it was good to see that she could learn. She just needed the right environment and the right person to motivate her. There is more about Emma's education in chapter 6.

After finding a suitable school for Emma, we turned our focus onto two courses of action. The first was to build a garden for Emma using the land we bought from Tony and Joan. Creating a garden from scratch with Emma especially in mind gave us new hope. It was hard work especially since neither Jeff nor I knew anything about gardening, but a marvellous therapy. The second requirement was to find therapies that might help Emma's development which is detailed in chapter 5.

Chapter 4

Our Rett Network

*Friendship is born at that moment when one
person says to another,
'What you too? I thought I was the only one.'*
C. S Lewis

Our membership of the RSAUK and the numerous benefits
it brought deserves a chapter to itself. Following Emma's
diagnosis in September 1994, we were desperate to find out
more about RS. The literature we received from RSAUK was
informative but we needed to share our experience more fully
with other RS parents.

We found Diane's address and telephone number in the
contact parents section of the *Rett News*. I telephoned Diane
who, with husband Brendan, had a six-year-old daughter
Hester with RS and a daughter Verity two years younger. We
had a chat for about 20 minutes about our experiences.

We visited Diane's family on Sunday 25th September. Hester
was pretty, a tall girl for her age. She walked well and stood
very erect. Jeff and I were amazed at how mobile she was,

considering her disability. Hester had involuntary hand movements and was sucking her fingers quite a lot, but other than that she appeared quite normal. She was unable to speak and Diane said that she usually greeted you by pulling your hair!

We talked a while about how Hester and Emma were getting on and the severity of their disability. Hester is at the high functioning end of the RS spectrum. She had never really had problems walking and could finger-feed herself quite well. Diane and Brendan had adapted their lifestyle to help Hester as much as possible. They continually had music playing in the background, which soothed Hester, and they had organised her bedroom and bathroom downstairs, so that she did not have to go upstairs much. Verity appeared very bright and seemed to know her sister's limitations.

We shared our experiences of discovering the decline of Hester's and Emma's skills, and the fight we had to go through to get a diagnosis. Our experiences were similar: the difficulty of convincing others and the shock of learning of the severity of the syndrome. Hester was an early developer – she could say a few words and paint before the age of one. Because she was so advanced, her regression was more noticeable. She was not diagnosed until she was nearly four.

Emma, as we have seen, was a late developer. She did not acquire many skills before the age of one and this made it difficult to detect her loss of skills. Her poor posture and lack of co-ordination were the more obvious signs of her illness.

One of the most useful and poignant pieces of advice Diane gave us was that we must not feel angry or bitter about having a special needs child. She quoted a poem which brought tears to my eyes. I could not remember the exact wording but it roughly meant that children with special needs were born to parents who can give them a lot of love and care. It was nature's way of protecting these children. In two weeks after diagnosis I had been asking the question 'Why me? What have I done to deserve this?' I found Diane's advice a great help. It gave me a lot of strength just thinking how much love and care other parents gave to their special needs children and how much I could learn from them.

Diane gave us a lot of support and practical advice. They told us that the diagnosis was a shock to them but they had come to terms with it in the last year. They said that once you accept it then you can get on with your life. We agreed on many things but one. Brendan seemed to think there was no hope of finding a cure for RS. He told me that I should not pin too much hope on a miracle cure. I could not agree with him. I believe there is hope – I believe that one day a cure will be found and that diagnosis screening will be possible. Perhaps I am being naive but I have to believe in it in order to keep my hopes alive. We stayed and had dinner with Diane's family. It was about nine o'clock when we left.

We kept in touch with Diane after our initial meeting. In September 1995, Diane asked us to a picnic with other Rett families in the Kent and Surrey area. It was raining and so we had to take our picnic to a Rett family's home. There we met

49

Judy and her daughter Sarah. They lived less than five minutes from where we used to live. In fact, Judy remembered that she had sat in the same waiting room with me nearly two years ago to see the paediatrician. She remembered me well because I was very sick that day – in fact I was suffering from food poisoning but I had insisted on taking Emma to her appointment.

After she received Sarah's diagnosis, Judy told me she had asked if there were any other families in the area that had a daughter with RS. She was told that there was but the hospital could not give her our name or address. She asked the hospital to check with us to see if we wanted contact. But we had heard nothing.

Judy and I became firm friends because we had so much in common. I like her directness, honesty and no-nonsense approach. She is a school teacher and her husband Paul is an accountant. They have a son Mark who is two years older than Sarah. Sarah was only two when she was diagnosed. She has beautiful long curly blonde hair. She seems to be smiling all the time. She has an interesting way of holding her hands as if she is playing the guitar.

Judy found it hard to accept Sarah's strange behaviour. She felt she could not love her because she could not understand her. The family had a hard time coming to terms with Sarah's condition. Mark did not understand why Sarah stopped doing the things she used to do and became frightened of meeting people with disabilities.

The diagnosis was devastating to the family but it helped them to make sense of Sarah's condition. They knew they had to do their best for Sarah. Paul decided to give up his job to look after Sarah. Understanding Sarah's condition really helped Judy to learn to love Sarah. Judy was interviewed by Simon Walker of *The Times* in October 2000. The feature was titled ' I've come to love her the way she is'. The diagnosis also helped Mark to understand why Sarah behaves the ways she does. He can now explain Sarah's condition to his friends. Mark organised a walk to raise money for RSAUK.

From 1995 until 1997, Judy and I belonged to a small local support group with about ten families from surrounding London boroughs. The families took it in turns to provide meeting facilities in their homes every three to four months. This group unfortunately stopped running after the death of one of the parents who organised it. A new group was formed when Judy was contacted by Sigi, a Rett mum who wanted to run a support group near Tunbridge Wells. With Sigi and her husband Ken's enthusiasm and efficiency, the group was well organised. Judy has now taken over organising this group with me as her right-hand woman! We meet up three times a year and the meetings are well attended. It is through this group that we build up good relationships with other parents.

Sigi's daughter Kim was diagnosed with RS at five. Sigi had to take Kim back to Germany for the diagnosis because she could not get any satisfactory explanations from doctors in England. Kim has pretty dark eyes and a mischievous sense of humour – she enjoys laughing at people's mistakes. Her younger brother Ian is very protective. Kim goes to a boarding school and comes home at weekends. Sigi takes Kim swimming once a fortnight and she loves it.

Charlotte is the same age as Emma but a few inches taller. She is the most mobile girl in the group. She can walk well and can walk up and down stairs, which is unusual for a Rett girl. Charlotte's mother Carolyn is devoted to her. Charlotte goes to a special school and she loves horse riding.

There is another Sarah in the group. She looks like a little angel : blonde hair, big blue eyes and a beautiful smile. It took Sarah's parents Kathy and Andrew a long time to get diagnosis for Sarah because her symptoms are atypical. She does not have the distinctive hand movements and her regression was not obvious.

Some members cannot come regularly because they have to come a long way. Occasionally, we have two RS women visitors from East Kent, or from other parts of London. The internet has made it possible for us to make friends with other Rett families outside our locality. We got to know the Foster family through a website for Stacey. Margaret has written a poignant story about her and she has kindly given me permission to include it here. This is the story of Margaret, her husband Ian and their beautiful daughter Stacey.

Stacey was born on 16th July 1983, their first child. The midwife told Margaret that she had a perfect little girl and

Margaret felt a rush of emotion as she held Stacey in her arms. She and Ian had wanted to have a child so much. But Stacey was not a contented baby. She would not breast feed and Margaret had to put her on a bottle.

She was achieving all her goals in the first year. At five weeks she smiled. The health visitor came to do her 12-month checkup and she was happy with Stacey's development. She was doing all the things that a normal one-year-old does: she would go and get the ball on request, bring her cup to Margaret for a refill and climb on the chair to see if her Daddy was coming home.

Soon after Stacey's first birthday Margaret began to wonder why she was not walking independently. At about 14 months, Stacey took a violent dislike to her cot. She would scream when she was put near it. The health visitor suggested putting Stacey in a bed instead but she would not stay in the bed. Margaret was advised to leave Stacey to scream, she would stop when she got tired. The screaming was heartbreaking and Margaret had to let Stacey come to her bed. The cuddling calmed Stacey and she went to sleep happily.

At 15 months, Stacey had her first fit and she had to be taken to hospital by ambulance. The doctor told Margaret that Stacey had had a febrile convulsion which is common in babies. She was told not to worry too much about it.

Margaret found it difficult to take Stacey to the mother's and toddler's group. As she sat watching the children play, she could not help comparing Stacey with other children. She seemed so much slower and it was upsetting to hear other mothers talking about the progress their children were making.

In March 1985, aged 20 months, Stacey was seen by a paediatrician in a local hospital. Margaret and Ian were given a lot of jargon about Stacey's condition and all Margaret could remember was the word 'damaged'. The paediatrician made an appointment for Stacey to have an EEG. Soon after the EEG, they took Stacey to the Child Development Centre to be assessed. The resident doctor asked a lot of detailed questions about Stacey's development history. Margaret asked her what level Stacey was at and she was told about 12 to 15 months. Ian asked whether she could catch up later but was told that she would never catch up and would have to go to a special school. Margaret was very angry with the doctor's dismissive attitude.

In December, at two and half years old, Stacey was diagnosed by the GP as having measles. A couple of days later she started to throw her legs out to the side. It looked really odd and as the days wore on it get worse. The GP referred Stacey to the hospital and she was put in the children's ward. The next day Stacey lost her ability to walk, and regressed to crawling.

In January 1986 Stacey had an appointment to see the genetics specialist at the Child Development Centre.

Margaret and Ian were hopeful that the doctor would be able to give a clear diagnosis. The doctor spent a lot of time going over Stacey's development history. He even checked the fingers and toes of Margaret, Ian and Stacey. At the end of the consultation, Margaret asked the doctor what he thought Stacey had. He said that he had an idea but was not prepared to say as he was not certain. At Margaret's insistence, he told them that he thought Stacey had RS. On the way home, it was snowing heavily. Margaret was so low the thought occurred to her that if the car crashed their suffering would be over. Margaret next joined a support group.

On 20th August 1987, a specialist in London finally confirmed it was RS. Stacey is now 26 years old. You can log on to the website (www.cleveleys.co.uk/staceyfoster) and read her full story.

As this chapter shows, the ways in which Rett Syndrome affects people are numerous, so the strategies to cope need a lot of thought.

Chapter 5

Looking for the Miracle

*There is no medicine like hope, no incentive so
great, and no tonic so powerful as expectation of
something tomorrow.*
O. S. Marden, author of motivational books

In November, 1994, I read an article in the Daily Mail about
a therapeutic treatment called Patterning which can help to
improve mobility in disabled children. I contacted the British
Institute for Brain Injured Children (BIBIC) in Bridgwater,
Somerset using the telephone number given in the paper.
There was huge response following the publication and we
managed to get Emma on the programme in March 1995.

The programme was intensive, long hours of doing exercises
and we needed a lot of help from our neighbours Joan,
Shanti, Janeki, Tamara and a volunteer Darren who later
became a friend. Emma hated the programme at first and
would not stop crying during the exercises. She did get used
to it after a few months. The progress was slow and we did
not see any noticeable improvement until after six months.
But the strain of spending time doing the exercises was

beginning to show especially at weekends when we wanted to spend time visiting family and friends and going for walks.

We continued with the programme for another six months before I decided to stop. There were two reasons for taking the decision. The first was the lack of time. My work started to get busy. Janeki and Tamara were also getting busy preparing for their school examinations. It was getting difficult to find time to do the patterning exercises. The second reason was we found a local school with a hydrotherapy pool that opened on Sundays. We took Emma swimming there and she loved it. I had not seen her giggling so much.

The patterning treatment has its supporters and detractors. Some people think it is a miracle cure and some think it is over-hyped physiotherapy. Most people who tried it found it to be of benefit. The treatment seemed to help at first, then the improvement would tail off. We found this to be true with Emma. It was worth the effort though and I was encouraged to find another treatment that could help Emma more. It took me to China.

In August 1996, during one of my shopping trips to Chinatown, I bought a Chinese magazine. Two articles enthralled. One was about the success stories of cranial acupuncture used in the GuangZhou Children's Hospital in GuangZhou city (formerly known as Canton) in Southern China. The other was about two Englishmen, Professor Brian Stratford and Jonathan Chamberlain setting up a charity called China Network for the Mentally Handicapped. Professor Stratford's work was based in GuangZhou, and Jonathan Chamberlain's work was based in Hong Kong.

I had constantly been on the lookout for treatments which could help Emma. I thought that she might benefit from acupuncture, Jeff agreed that we should give it a try. Finding information about the treatment and the hospital, however, was extremely difficult. I contacted the Chinese magazine and they passed me from department to department and no one seemed able to track down the journalist who wrote the article. The Chinese Embassy was not much help either.

My parents had made plans to visit China in March the following year. I thought I could go with them and use the opportunity to find the hospital during our holiday. In September, I enrolled into a local evening class to learn to speak Mandarin as a preparation for my holiday to China.

In March 1997, Jeff, Emma and I set off for our two week holiday in Hong Kong and China. The plan was to stay a few days with my parents in Hong Kong, then go to Shenzhen and GuangZhou for a few days. During the visit to GuangZhou, I would leave the organised guided tour for half a day to find the hospital and then rejoin them later. I failed to find the address of the children's hospital. In the end, it was my sister Jane who found an article in the *South China Morning Post* about Professor Stratford and Maureen Stratford's work in the GuangZhou Children's Hospital. I contacted the Stratfords and they made an appointment for me to meet Dr Lee at the hospital to discuss Emma receiving cranial acupuncture on a Thursday afternoon.

On Tuesday, we set off for China. The first stop was Shenzhen, China's first Special Economic Zone. We visited a theme park called the China Folk Culture Villages. We took a walk in a park near the hotel after dinner and there we had an unpleasant experience. An elderly woman with a young woman walked towards us. As they walked near us, the elderly woman put her hand out to touch Emma and said what a pretty girl she was. The young woman quickly pulled the elderly woman away from Emma and said to her 'She has polio'. Such ignorance about disability is common in China.

On Thursday, we moved on to GuangZhou. While my parents and the other members of our group visited the zoo, Jeff, Emma and I took a taxi to the hospital. We asked for Professor Stratford at the reception and were met by Maureen Stratford a few minutes later. She took us to a room in the Mentally Retarded Rehabilitation Unit to meet Dr Lee, who was in charge. I explained Emma's condition to Dr Lee and asked her whether she thought the treatment would work on her. She told me that the treatment worked well with children who suffered brain injuries after birth but not so well on children with genetic disorders. I was disappointed by her reply but was glad that she was honest with me. I then asked her whether it would do Emma any harm to have the treatment and she said it was unlikely to harm her. Jeff and I could not make a decision there and then and we thought it would be best to decide when back in England. After much consideration back at home, we decided to give it a try.

I managed to get four months off work between November 1997 and February 1998. On Saturday, 1st November 1997 Jeff saw Emma and me off at the airport. Thanks to the travel sickness medicine, Emma slept most of the time and when she was awake she was well-behaved. I was given help by the air hostess on the trip between the plane and the baggage reclaim. The most difficult part was getting the luggage and Emma through customs on arrival in Hong Kong – I had to hold onto Emma with one hand and to steer the trolley containing over 40kg of luggage with the other.

We stayed in my brother John's apartment in Hong Kong for the night. The next day, Jane went up to Guangzhou with us on the train. A taxi dropped us off on the side of the road opposite the hospital. It was a nightmare crossing that road to the hospital. We found that cars do not give way to pedestrians, they just weave between them.

We arrived at the hospital about 1pm. I told the woman at the reception that we wanted to see Dr Lee and she told us to report to the nurses' station on the first floor. There was no one at the nurses' station. In fact, the whole place looked deserted. Eventually I heard some noises from a room. I knocked on the door to see whether anyone could help. Maureen Stratford, wife of Professor Stratford, opened the door. Inside there were Professor Stratford, Hannah and Kerry who were teachers, and Frances and Richard who were interpreters.

Maureen welcomed us in. I asked her where everyone was. She told me everyone was having a siesta – the whole unit closed between twelve noon and half past two in the afternoon. Emma started to moan because she was hungry. Maureen told us to leave the luggage in their room and go out and get some lunch.

When we came back after lunch, the whole place was buzzing with activity. Parents with children were sitting in the treatment room. I could hear children crying. One of the children came out into the corridor with needles all over his head, arm and legs. He gave Jane quite a fright as she did not know what cranial acupuncture treatment involved. We were seen by a nurse. There were numerous forms to fill in. I had to give Emma a Chinese name and my maiden name for the ease of registration, so for the next four months Emma was to be known as Chan Eai Man. Part of the admission process involved having Emma's weight, height and temperature measured. Emma dropped the thermometer and it broke. The nurse told me that I had to pay 10 yens straight away because they needed the money to buy a new one.

When the check-in was over, we collected our luggage from Maureen's office and moved into our allocated room. All in-patients from abroad or Hong Kong had to be given special grade rooms. Ours was a large room with two single beds. There was a television, small fridge and our own bathroom. I was pleased to find that we had a modern toilet. It is true that no matter what language you speak money talks.

After helping us to get settled in, Jane left to return to Hong Kong. The next day, Tuesday, I woke up quite late, still having a problem adjusting to local time. While I was getting Emma ready for the treatment, I could hear children crying down the corridor. When I took a look I saw a number of parents with their children waiting outside the treatment room. At nine o'clock, I took Emma to see Professor Zue for her initial assessment. Professor Zue was the man who developed the cranial acupuncture treatment for children with neurological disorders. He was between 50 and 60, a little abrupt, but very observant. He noticed that Emma's head was smaller than normal – a fact that is not apparent to most people. I told him about Emma's condition and showed him the translated description of RS. Although Professor Zue was not familiar with RS, he had a good understanding of Emma's problems. As he was taking notes and writing down Emma's treatment plan, I noticed a crowd of people were gathering outside the room. Some of them were poking their heads through the open door and window.

I could hear them saying things like that is the girl from England, and she has pretty eyes. I found it quite distracting with all that noise in the background while trying my best to explain things in Mandarin. Eventually, the assessment finished and Professor Zue told me to take Emma to the treatment room. The treatment room was large with a long table, chairs and a television. Quite a few children had already been given their treatment, sitting there with needles sticking out of their heads, arms and legs. Some of them were crying.

I sat down with Emma and waited for someone to give her treatment. As we waited, we saw some children having needles inserted into them. Some would cry and some would struggle. One little boy had to be held down by three adults. When it was Emma's turn, she took it calmly, no tears, she did not bat an eyelid. All the mothers and grandmothers marvelled at Emma's calmness and bravery. They told their children and grandchildren to look at the brave little girl. I knew it was not bravery. It was all to do with Emma's lack of awareness of danger and impaired sense of pain which are symptoms of RS.

Emma had to sit still for half an hour with the needles. The needles had to be turned 360 degrees every ten minutes. She was very good and sat there watching a cartoon. When she was sitting still, I had a chance to talk to other people who were full of questions. They were curious about Emma's condition. I had to explain RS to them which was not an easy task since they kept telling me that it may have something to do with my eating the wrong type of food when I was pregnant. It is a common belief that this causes disability.

The other children in the treatment room had different disabilities but the acupuncture treatment they received was similar. The only noticeable differences were the number of needles and some had electrodes attached to the needles. Most of them cried when the needles were inserted but they calmed down after a while. It was a very upsetting experience sitting in a room with these children suffering pain and fear. I found out from the parents that most of the children come to the day clinic for treatment; only a few stayed in the hospital. Some of them had to travel a long way.

Later that day, Emma had a massage and two injections. The doctor who gave Emma the massage was a student doctor called Dr Yin. He was good with Emma and she took to him straight away. Emma was given two injections on her back close to her spine. I tried to find out what was in the injections but the nurse would not tell me.

In the evening, I took Emma to the TV room to watch television with the other children and meet the other mothers and grandmothers. All the children staying in the rehabilitation unit were from fairly well-off families. The less well-off children came to the day clinic. I was moved by the devotion to children I saw. Before I came to China, I had a preconceived idea that in China most disabled children were abandoned, living in institutions without love or care. The most difficult part was the stigma associated with disability – a shameful experience for the family. The only consolation was (if it can be considered a consolation) that the couple could apply to have a second child, an exception to the rule of China's One Child Policy.

Looking after a disabled child in England is difficult but looking after a disabled child in China is ten times worse. There are few schools for either mentally or physically disabled children. Most of them are kept at home. There was no assistance from the government at all in terms of financial help or provision of health and social services. There are few charities or self-help groups to support the family.

The children in the unit were cared for by their families. Very often, the mother would stay with the child during the treatment period. If she ran out of leave, a grandmother or another female relative would come to help out. Most people are employed by state-owned organisations, and so most mothers could return to their work after taking time off to look after their children.

Although I missed the home comforts, such as having a bath, I settled in quickly. The other mothers and the grandmothers were helpful. They took me round to the local market and helped me to buy some cooking utensils. Emma had a few problems with food and she missed her videos. She was used to having toast and cereal for breakfast. I managed to get some cornflakes but I could not get a toaster. Jane brought me a toaster from Hong Kong and the woman in the next room went with me to buy a video machine.

Emma was happy again with the food she was familiar with and she could watch her favourite videos. The other children also enjoyed watching Emma's videos even though they had no English. They loved imitating the movements.

A few days after we arrived, Maureen arranged for Emma to join the hospital playgroup. Emma attended for an hour in the morning and an hour in the afternoon. The playgroup was for children who stay at the rehabilitation unit. Emma's teacher was Hannah, brought up in Scotland by a Chinese father and Scottish mother. Hannah was a Psychology graduate who had wanted to work in China for a few years. She had some problems with Emma initially before she got to know her ways. Emma would close her eyes when she was not interested in doing something such as sorting bricks by colours and she got bored after a while. Hannah thought she was tired all the time. Emma also played up by pushing all the toys onto the floor when she was not getting enough attention. Once Hannah worked out what Emma enjoyed doing, they got on well. While Emma attended the playgroup I had the time to go shopping or prepare meals.

Emma's daily programme consisted of half an hour acupuncture and an hour in the playgroup. In the afternoon, she had half an hour massage and an hour in the playgroup. There was a lot of time to spare, so I decided to train Emma to feed herself using a spoon, suck through a straw and walk up and down the stairs. These were the things I had tried unsuccessfully to do back home due to the lack of time with her and the different methods of feeding and drinking at school.

For teaching her to feed herself with a spoon, I used a wrist strap to secure a spoon with a thick handle to her hand, filled the spoon with food and encouraged her to move the spoon to her mouth by herself. It was a frustrating experience for both Emma and me. Very often, the food would fall out of the spoon before it got to her mouth. Also, Emma closed her mouth too early. She had her mouth wide open while she was moving the spoon towards her mouth but she closed it before the spoon got there. I resolved the first problem by mixing food with sticky rice or mashed potato. It took Emma about two months to get the timing of opening and closing her mouth right.

Teaching her to suck from a straw was impossible until I found cartons of fruit juice in a supermarket. The first few times, I had to squeeze the carton to squirt the drink into her mouth. After a while she got the hang of it. Teaching Emma to walk up and down the stairs proved to be a difficult task due to her impaired sense of distance and after a few weeks, my arms and shoulders were aching and I had to give up.

There were flowers and fish tanks on every floor but there were not enough walking frames or wheelchairs for children with walking difficulties. The whole of GuangZhou city ran like that – not enough traffic lights and pedestrian crossings, but the parks were beautiful. The hospital also suffered frequent power cuts.

Professor Stratford and Maureen set up the playgroup at the hospital to help the children to learn. There are self-help groups for parents with disabled children and training materials on different types of disabilities such as Down's Syndrome, cerebral palsy and autism for teachers, doctors and nurses. While we were there, Hannah and Kerry ran the playgroup with Maureen. The parents' club met once a month to share experiences and view training materials. A video in English was often shown which Frances translated into Chinese. The Stratfords' work attracted a lot of interest from the teaching and medical professions all over China. Nearly every week, we had visitors from different places. One of the things that I found annoying was that the children's learning activities were disrupted when visitors arrived. They had to put on a show, sitting together singing songs.

Weekends were very quiet. Most of the mothers and children went home to be with their families. Two families usually stayed at the weekend. Ton Ton, a little boy with cerebral palsy and his mother, and Qing Sing, a little boy with Down's Syndrome and his grandmother. My sister Jane came to visit us every other weekend. We often went out to a park. Ton Ton's mother and Qing Sing's grandmother were reluctant to go out. Ton Ton's mother was worried about not being able to carry Ton Ton, so I lent him Emma's pushchair. Qing Sing's grandmother was worried about people staring at Qing Sing, so I told her not to be bothered by ignorant people. They came out with us and had a great time. Ton Ton and Qing Sing could not wait for our next outing.

The treatment did not seem to have much effect on Emma for the first few weeks. After about a month, I noticed Emma started to feel pain when needles were inserted into her. It was as much pain for me as for her to watch her receiving her treatment. Gradually I began to see some improvements in her hands, they were less rigid and she was not biting them as much as she did. I thought the treatment must have improved her sense of touch and she was not dribbling as much as she used to, but there was no improvement in her legs.

I asked Dr Lee why there was no improvement in her legs. She explained that the parts that were closest to the head would get better first, then improvements would slowly filter down to the rest of the body. This appeared to be the case with other children. Leg problems certainly seemed to take longest to improve.

Emma became frightened of nurses who wore pink uniforms. She associated these with the acupuncture. The only person in uniform that Emma was pleased with was Lan who came to do the beds. She was entertaining and always smiling and Emma loved to hear her sing even though she did not understand a word. Sometimes Lan would get Emma to help her push her trolley around the unit and she would bring her 10 year-old son to play with Emma.

I started to feel homesick in December despite Jeff telephoning nearly every other day and having made a few friends. The worst time was Christmas. Maureen and Hannah organised a Christmas party for the children. They enjoyed the food and the games even though they did not fully understand the meaning of Christmas. Emma's teacher in England, Elaine, sent us a big parcel containing a card signed by all the teachers and children and small presents from the class. I was touched by their kindness.

I could not help noticing that there were a large number of Westerners with Chinese babies. They had come to China to adopt the abandoned baby girls. This appeared to be the perfect solution to the abandoned babies problem. Childless couples get to have a baby and China gets rid of its unwanted female babies, but I am not convinced that this is a good solution. It does not stop people killing or abandoning female babies or solve the problem of an unbalanced number of males and females in the population.

Lack of basic facilities such as wheelchairs and walking frames were real problems for families with disabilities. Some of the things that I brought from England really fascinated them: the pelican bib, the toilet training ring, spoons with thick handles, jigsaw puzzles with pegs. I could see these things could be of real help to them. My mother was coming back to Hong Kong for Chinese New Year. I asked her to buy ten of each item. When Chinese New Year came, I gave them out as presents.

The unit closed for one week over the Chinese New Year period in February 1998. Emma and I went to stay with my parents in Hong Kong. It was a welcome relief for Emma not having to receive acupuncture treatment. I enjoyed my stay in Hong Kong very much. It was the first time I had had a proper bath in three months and the first Chinese New Year I had had in Hong Kong since we moved to England 25 years before.

We went back to GuangZhou after the Chinese New Year at the beginning of February. The leaflets for the Stratfords' charity China Network for the Mental Handicap had been printed and Emma was on the cover. They told me that they were going to produce a quarterly magazine for the parents' club and they asked me to write an article about Emma.

On our last day in the hospital, all the children and mothers in the unit came to say goodbye and brought us presents. Jane and my Mum came to help us to take our luggage back to Hong Kong.

Some of the improvements made in China such as less drooling and the ability to make a wider range of sounds faded a few months after we came back. Emma managed, however, to retain the skills to feed herself, sucking through a straw and keeping her back straight.

The most valuable thing I gained from the trip was my closer relationship with Emma. We spent so much time together, it helped me to get to know her better. I learned more about China in four months than I ever learned from books and newspapers. I was saddened by the way disabled people and unwanted baby girls were treated. I was dismayed by the bureaucracy and inefficiency I saw in the hospital and outside but I felt uplifted by the parents' determination to make a better life for their disabled children. The trip also gave me an opportunity to make a small contribution to help others.

We kept in touch with the Stratfords and Hannah. The Special Children's Club went from strength to strength. They helped to form new clubs in other cities in China. They also opened another clinic in the east side of GuangZhou. Hannah stayed in China for another year and then came back to England to study for a postgraduate degree in education.

I believe the nurse's indiscretion also fuelled Dr Stratford's determination to make people understand disability and learn to help sufferers. He wrote two books on Down's Syndrome and he became the chairman of the Down's Syndrome Association in the UK and the principal advisor to the Hong Kong Down's Syndrome Association.

With funding form the Keswick Foundation in Hong Kong, the Stratfords set up a club for parents with disabled children in GuangZhou, producing training material and giving lectures on different types of disability. The Stratfords have given hope to parents with disabled children in GuangZhou and they have advised the medical professionals on how to work with the families of disabled children. In 2001 they were both awarded the OBE for their contribution to working with disabled children and their families. In 2004, the GuangZhou Municipal Government conferred on the Stratfords the GuangZhou Friendship Award to honour their work for the city.

Chapter 6

Educating Emma

*Exceptional human beings must be given
exceptional educational treatment, treatment
which takes into account their special difficulties.
Further, we can show that despite
abnormality, human beings can fulfil their social
role within the community, especially if they find
understanding, love and guidance.*
Hans Asperger, Austrian paediatrician and
psychologist

From Elaine, Emma's first teacher at the special unit, we
learned how important it was to have someone who can
recognise Emma's ability. But even the most competent
teacher can have a problem getting through to Emma. It is
vital that the teachers know about RS and how to bring out
the best of her abilities. The extract below from the booklet
An Introduction to Rett Syndrome produced by RSAUK
explains how to educate girls with RS.

*Girls who have RS have great aptitude to learn and
can progress, particularly when highly motivated*

to do so. The girls with RS will need a school placement where there are facilities and expertise to manage their education, therapy and care as a holistic and continuous process. While it is most likely that this will be provided in a local special school, there is no doubt that the girls who have RS are very sociable and really enjoy activities with their more able peers.

The school should have a clear understanding of the girls' development needs and offer a curriculum designed to take on board the girls' profound learning difficulties while offering meaningful and relevant experience. Successful teaching also depends on understanding the barriers which inhibit the girls' learning – their delayed response to stimuli, their hand dysfunction and stereotypical movements, their apraxia and poor motor control.

Learning tasks should be broken down into small, achievable steps relevant to each girl. While accurate and frequent assessments monitor her needs and abilities, particular attention should be paid to developing communication, cognitive, perceptual and physical skills. Good diet management, attention to her personal care and involvement in leisure activities will all support the integrated process of the girls' education.

Emma goes to a local school for children with severe learning difficulties. The school has wide expertise in special needs and they also have expertise in teaching children with RS. It offers a curriculum that includes adaptations of subjects on the national curriculum, plus therapies such as hydrotherapy, horse riding, physiotherapy and speech therapy. Subjects are adapted in a creative way to suit the children's ability. For example, instead of learning about faraway places such as America or Africa in Geography, children will be taught things around them that they can relate to. Special equipment such as computer switches (specially adapted devices for activating computers, or other electronic machines) and a Starlight (multi-sensory) room are used to encourage children to communicate.

This is an extract from Emma's school report (July 2002) which gives an insight into the work Emma did when she was 11.

English and Communication

Emma is able to give good eye contact when she finds the context or activity stimulating. Generally, she prefers to look at and study faces rather than objects or pictures. I have seen her demonstrate her best looking skills, that is, looking at the materials with which she is working, when working with soapy water in a one-to-one interaction with an adult and similarly, when exploring freshly cut grass and cotton wool. She looks very well at a candle in a darkened room and at the bubble tube in the Starlight room. Emma clearly finds some materials and media de-motivating and she makes this known by moving her hands or by sharply withdrawing them, mouthing her hands, adopting a 'floppy' posture or closing her eyes.

Emma gives clear indications of motivation and 'like' but we are as yet not consistently able to mould these responses into a clear gesture for 'more' to encourage her to be more active than passive in interactions. This, alongside developing her ability to take turns, will remain a strong focus.

Emma's listening skills are quite difficult to assess but she will respond with a turn of the head or eye contact to her name when stated clearly. Naturally, she has voices that she responds to better and it is important that she is given opportunities to develop her communication skills with those adults and peers she finds most comfortable. Emma will not always respond actively to our music sessions but has clearly demonstrated that she is able to hear a beat or rhythm by spontaneously tapping her fingers on her tray. She has done this consistently to livelier beats.

Emma has shown that she is able to use a Big Mack switch to say 'Good morning' but she may often hit the switch erratically and repetitively if at all and it is debatable as to how motivating she finds this. I feel a better alternative needs to be explored. Generally, I am not convinced that Emma has consistently demonstrated an understanding of cause and effect.

Mathematics
Emma is introduced to numbers through games, songs and

stories and her concentration is generally good. She reacts well to familiar songs and her face will light up with recognition. Her favourite song is 'This Old Man'.

Emma continues to enjoy her weekly sessions in the Starlight room, where we encourage her to use switches appropriately to activate the equipment and to concentrate on the equipment. We also expect her to relax a little, something she can find difficult and she is encouraged to lie down on the waterbed and enjoy the fibre optic cascade, using her hands and voluntarily taking them out of her mouth and purposefully using them. We also allow Emma a time in the Starlight room to walk around safely, looking and moving freely between the different pieces of equipment.

Science

Our work this term has centred around 'Ourselves and other animals'. Much of this topic has focussed on the senses and what they enable us to do. Emma has demonstrated that she is motivated to look at shiny, bright media and to listen to classical music, especially Mozart. It would be interesting to have a tape of familiar voices, maybe reading a short story, and analyse how she responds to this. We undertook a taste and smell survey. Emma demonstrated clearly that she liked the taste of banana, jam, baked bean juice, sugar, brown bread and basil: she did this simply by taking and eating more when offered. Emma did not like the taste of celery, marmite, salad cream or salt and indicated this by pushing away or spitting out. She did appear to like the smell of celery, banana, basil and marmite and generally indicated this with a smile and a look at the adult holding the food.

Emma has enjoyed walking in the wooded area of the school grounds, she has indicated this by walking with greater purpose and by looking around at her environment. She has looked at mice and giant snails and was reported to have observed their movement closely, touching the snails. She has happily helped to collect grass and flowers for a wormery.

Looking back through class records, it is evident that the most purposeful avenue for Emma to pursue in Science is through investigation. We encourage her to interact with and explore her world in a proactive, meaningful way.

Geography
We have been studying 'Leisure time' and have looked at and experienced many of the wide variety of ways the children and staff spend their free time. Emma was not impressed with the drawings and sketches. She was taken with the piano playing adult but again not so impressed by the adult showing her how to do tapestry work. Generally the children make it clear that watching TV is a good way to spend one's leisure time. Emma also makes it quite clear that she likes to go for walks and enjoys being outdoors (when shown pictures of gardens and large houses she got quite animated).

Weather around the world was a topic in which Emma enjoyed being helped to dress up to simulate different weather conditions. Emma was singularly unimpressed at wearing cold weather clothing; hats, gloves and scarves, giving the *adult with her a very odd look. It really is so good that we can tell just by looking at Emma's face what she thinks of the activity.*

History
Emma has had plenty of experience of artefacts and resources based around the themes of 'People who help us' and 'Victorian Britain'. Emma has enjoyed dressing up as a policeman and as a Victorian child. This term, Emma has been contributing to a 'Special Book' in the context of the Queen's Golden Jubilee. We also looked at the events around the Jubilee and the World Cup in the newspapers.

The 2002 report shows the difficulties that the teachers had with understanding and communicating with Emma. She can be quite a challenge to teachers who do not know her as shown in an article about Emma written by a new teacher in the school newsletter in the summer term of 2002.

If Emma was a wine, the label might suggest she was 'dry, complex with lively, fruity spark.' What an enigma Emma is. She has the sort of face that can light up your whole day when she smiles or make you feel an inch high when giving you one of her stares! Happily, I am getting more smiles than stares these days (though she always smiles at Carol, Bridget and Gill) and it is clear that Emma's sense of humour is not only well-formed and well-judged but can also veer on the side of mischievous – never are her smiles wider for me than when she is pirouetting on one foot, getting me to take all her weight and pretending she can't stand up. She is a ray of sunshine and a soothing presence in amongst a squadron of boys.

Over the years, Emma has made some improvements in communicating her needs. Also the introduction of the Smartboard has made teaching and communicating with Emma easier as shown in her 2009 school report.

Emma is a member of a mixed ability class of students in the Further Education (FE) Department age between 16 and 17 years old. The class is staffed by one teacher and three teaching assistants. Students follow a developmental curriculum, which is fully differentiated to meet their needs. In addition, Emma has Individual Education Programme targets for English and Communication, Numeracy, Personal, Social and Health Education (PSHE) and Independence/ICT. Emma has access to a number of specialist facilities including a sunken trampoline, hydrotherapy; pool work based learning resources, a multi-sensory room, cooking and life skills facilities

Ability Literacy/Communication Sessions
During the sessions Emma participated and engaged in interactive story and poetry telling. She enjoyed both Legends and a sensory version of A Christmas Carol, responding to a range of stimuli, sensory objects and activities. Using her established means of communication, Emma demonstrated her enjoyment. For example, she smiled in response to images displayed on the Smartboard, vocalised joyfully when a parachute was wafted above her or giggled when tickled with

a feather duster. Emma responded generally positively to interactive poems and especially enjoyed auditory elements. She listened intently to poem rhythms being tapped out using wooden sticks. Emma's communicative responses often depended on her general wellbeing and on auditory input.

Interactive story telling and poetry sessions have created opportunities for Emma to communicate using switches. She made a great effort at activating a small jelly bean switch to build a story or ask for a turn.

This half term, the group has begun work on interactive poetry. Here, Emma will look at the Smartboard, which has a pre-loaded story and at the appropriate stage she will be encouraged to respond by touching a switch that has a pre-recorded sentence or word on it. Emma has worked well in this situation and does respond to the prompts from the story. She does need some adult support, but has been responding by pushing the switch button as well as smiling.

Currently we are being trained in the use of our new sensory room; we will use this as a further stimulus for Emma's communication skills in the coming months. Emma has clear responses to situations that she likes and situations and stimulation that she does not like. Emma will vocalise and move her body excitedly when she is enjoying a particular event. When Emma dislikes something, she can be seen to visibly have a grimace on her face and/or she will look away.

This year we have been involved with a production of Oliver

Twist, an interactive storytelling adaptation written by Keith Parks. This involved Emma in a range of call and response activities in conjunction with her peers. Emma used a switch with adult help and was very excited when the switch was pressed and this triggered a number of responses. The whole experience seemed to stimulate Emma and she would smile and on occasions verbalise.

We have also had sessions with Tim and Tom from Mousetrap Theatre. This is a musical experience where students join in with musical stories. Emma really enjoyed this and was excited when her name was sung. This kind of stimulation is important for Emma as it seems to engage her fully with what is happening in her school day.

Ability Numeracy Sessions
This year, work in numeracy included anticipation and counting games, making instant desserts as well as simple biscuits. Emma made a great effort at reaching out for balls whilst playing target games. She showed a clear preference for a bumpy ball and would often indicate her choice by decisive-eye-pointing. Emma used both her hands to tap and to touch a ball she liked. She also managed to track a rolling bell ball or skittles being knocked over. Emma displayed her anticipation skills in construction games. She smiles broadly on hearing 1, 2, 3 rote counting before knocking a block tower over. Whilst working on preparing instant desserts, Emma was encouraged to operate a food mixer using a small jelly bean switch. Once started off, she would tap the switch independently to turn the mixer on and off. She also used her

eye-pointing skills to choose between two dessert options and loved testing chocolate Angel Delight, opening her mouth to indicate her desire for more and smiling occasionally.

PSHE (Personal, Social and Health Education)
In PSHE Emma has been involved with staff in massage and some music therapy. Emma has been looking at the Smartboard screen which is pre-loaded with moving colour schemes. Whilst Emma is listening to the music she is actively following patterns displayed on the Smartboard.

This year Emma had two visits to Wood Lodge. During this time she has stayed overnight with her peers. Emma has had the opportunity to help with the preparation of the meals. Here staff use hand over hand techniques to enable her to participate in daily living skills, for example to cut up vegetables or use a Hoover. Emma also had the opportunity to see the musical Lion King in London. Emma enjoyed this experience and she was visibly excited during the performance.

Work Based Learning
This term we are involved in a mini-enterprise project that involved Emma and her peers producing items that we can sell at school. Emma helped to make these items using hand over hand techniques and was fully integrated into the project which also involved painting and cooking. Emma used switches and hand over hand techniques to achieve some of the activities: for example with adult help she was able to make some of the patterns of the glass vases. This sometimes

83

proved a little difficult, but she experienced some success. Emma reacts well to this type of creative activity, she is happy to cooperate with the adult and is often seen to be concentrating for short periods of time on her hand whilst it is working on different aspects of the project.

ASDAN (Award Scheme Development and Accreditation Network)

This year along with her peers, Emma has been involved in the ASDAN 'Towards Independence' accreditation scheme. Here Emma has been working on a topic that involves knowing yourself and your school and home environment. Emma, along with adult help, has investigated her personal features. She used mirrors to explore this part of the topic. She enjoyed this and was always smiling when she looked into the mirror.

We have also introduced Emma to her complete school environment. She has explored both the old and new parts of the building. She has responded well to this section of the topic and staff have been able to elicit a response from her when they are talking about certain areas. She responded to the nurses' station and she obviously enjoys being with our nursing staff. She responded positively to the trampoline area and the school pool.

Physical Development

Emma has regular trampoline sessions and she really responds well to these and is visibly excited about the prospect of being out of her chair and is quite vocal when *she is lifted out of her chair onto the trampoline. The motion involved is very stimulating for her and she responds with vocal excitement, her eyes light up and her smile is enormous. Emma has regular sessions and these are important to her as it gives her a chance to move her legs without putting pressure on her joints. She enjoys these sessions and is always smiling when she is in the pool.*

We understand that Emma's education does not just take place in school. She can learn from all the things around her. We try to take Emma out at weekends as much as possible. Emma enjoys going out to farms to look at the animals. She also loves going to visit shopping centres, gardens and buildings of interest. We find the communication book useful in exchanging information with her teachers on Emma's daily activities in school and at home. Emma is now 18 and she has one more year at school and then she will attend a college of further education. At the time of writing, we are still uncertain whether the local council will provide funding for her further education.

Chapter 7

Emma in my Dreams

*Dreams are an outlet for the fulfilment of our
deepest wishes and desires.*
Sigmund Freud

I love films and their dream-like quality. My dreams of Emma
are like films – they give me the means to escape from reality
and to enjoy a new kind of life. Not only night-time dreams
but also daytime dreams help me to feel more complete. I
have known orphans who have provided themselves with
parents in their dreams.

Weeks before our visit to China, I had started having this
recurring dream. I dreamt that I was outside a school gate
waiting for Emma. When the bell rang, the children came
rushing out of the classrooms. Emma was the first one out.
She ran towards me with a picture in her hand calling
'Mummy, Mummy. Look, I have drawn a picture of you, me
and Daddy.' She held the picture up in front of me. It was a
picture of a woman, a girl and a man in matchstick style with
the sun and a tree in the background – a typical child's
drawing. I smiled and told her that it was a lovely picture. I

rolled the picture up, took Emma's hand and made our way home. She talked excitedly about her day in school while we walked home.

I spoke to my neighbour Joan about this and she told me that she also had dreamt about Emma. She dreamt that she took Emma and her grandchildren to the seaside. They all had a good time playing on the beach. One of her grandchildren wanted to have an ice-cream and Emma said 'I want an ice-cream too'. Joan told me that it is common to dream about people with disability having a normal life. Joan's husband Tony used to dream about being able to walk, run and do all the things that a normal person would do. In a sense, Tony and I were both living a nightmare and the dreams we had were cruel fantasies of what should have been.

In the weeks leading up to Emma's tenth birthday, I started having a different dream about Emma. Jeff had bought me a mobile phone for my birthday, three weeks before Emma's birthday. I was eager to try out all the functions – phone book, text message, alarm, screen savers and games. But I kept being interrupted by people ringing up about Emma's party. Joan wanted to know what decoration to put on the birthday cake, Grace wanted to know what food I wanted for the party, other parents wanted to know what Emma would like for her birthday present. I really wished I knew what Emma wanted, so I did not have to wrack my brain to think. I looked at this shiny new phone in my hand and suddenly remembered the advertising logo: 'Who would you like to have a one-to-one with?' A mad idea came to my head – what if I could have a one-to-one with Emma by phone? She could answer all my questions.

I felt sad that Emma's tenth birthday was almost here, I did not even know who she would like to invite to her party, where she would like to have the party, what presents she would like to have, what she would like on her birthday cake, what she would like to wear, what music she would like to have, what games she would like to play?

That night, I had a dream about Emma ringing me on my mobile from her school friend Victoria's house asking me if she could go shopping with Victoria to spend her birthday money. I asked her what she was going to buy. She said she was going to buy make-up, jewellery and clothes. I told her that she should not buy make-up because she is too young. We started an argument with Emma accusing me of being too boring and old fashioned and me accusing her of being careless with money. I got so angry with her that I switched the phone off.

I began to ask myself many other questions. What does Emma think of me? Does she think I am too strict with her, incessantly telling her not to bite her hands or grind her teeth? Does she think I am boring and old-fashioned? Does she think I do not spend enough time with her? Does she like the food I cook? Does she get upset because I could not go to her sports days or school play? Does she like the clothes and shoes we buy her? Does she like the way we decorate her bedroom? So many questions I do not have answers for.

Whenever I dreamt about Emma, she was always normal. She was so different to the real Emma. These dreams made me think what Emma might have been. What would Emma be like if she were 'normal'?

This is the Emma of my dreams. She mixes in well at Cara's first birthday party, crawling and playing with other children. After her first birthday, she starts to say longer words such as bottle and telephone. She surprises Jeff's parents by calling them Nan and Gran. She loves reading books, especially ones with colourful pictures.

When Emma becomes able to walk around on her own, she is eager to explore the house. We have to rearrange the furniture in the house so that she would not trip, we have to put away the ornaments and anything like scissors that may cause harm, block all the electric sockets with plastic plugs, and put stoppers to prevent drawers from being opened. We have to make sure all household cleaning substances and chemicals used for gardening are kept away from her. We also have to make sure we keep her away from pens and crayons to stop her drawing all over the walls. We have to put up stair gates to stop her going up or down stairs on her own.

During her holiday in Hong Kong, her lovely smile charms all those who met her. She learns to point at things, and toddled to places. She enjoys the attention of my family and friends. She enjoys the visit to Ocean Park, watching the dolphins, seals and killer whales perform. She is fascinated by the visit to the temple at Lan-Tau island, the smell of burning incense, the huge statue of the Buddha, and the chanting of the monks.

At the nursery, she makes friends with other children, she becomes more socially aware, learns to share toys with other children and to take turns. As well as social skills, she learns self-help skills, singing and painting. Often, she comes home singing songs she learns in her own style with missing words and completely out of tune. Jeff and I have great fun playing name that tune with Emma's singing. At the end of each term, she brings home a large collection of her art work which fills up the garage.

Like all children, my dream Emma has tantrums when she cannot get her own way or the attention she wants. She cries or spends hours sulking. She sometimes rebels when asked to do things that she does not want to do. Occasionally, she becomes spiteful and says things like 'I don't like this' or 'I hate you'. She sometimes becomes jealous of other children because they have things that she does not. When she gets older, she learns to manipulate to get things she wants.

When she learns to talk properly, it is difficult to stop her. She asks all sorts of questions, why is this, what is that , how do you do this? She comes home with all sorts of stories about her day, talking about her friends and teachers. She jumps at the chance of answering the phone every time it rings and bores the hapless caller with her ramble. She makes us laugh or cringe by using inappropriate words and phrases she picks up from her friends or television. She drives everyone mad by telling them what is going to happen next.

Emma becomes attached to the teddy bear Jeff bought her when she was a baby. She insists on taking it everywhere, to the nursery and on holiday. She loves the large collection of soft toys given to her by friends and relatives. She brings them out to show off to her friends when they come to visit. When she gets older, she moves on to the ultimate girl's toy – Barbie Doll. She has a collection of different sizes of Barbie, and her vast selection of costumes. She spends hours brushing Barbie's hair and changing her clothes.

One day, Emma tells us she wants a pet. This triggers a great debate about what to have and who is going to look after it. Jeff does not want to have a dog because it is a chore having to take it for a walk every day. Emma was allowed to have a hamster. Jeff and I gave her a lengthy talk about the responsibilities of looking after a pet. The first few months, Emma fed and cleaned the hamster with great enthusiasm. She loses interest after a while; Jeff and I end up looking after it.

Emma loves Christmas. Each year, she cannot wait to see the pretty Christmas lights, meeting Father Christmas, and going to parties. She insists on helping to decorate the Christmas tree, writing out Christmas cards and wrapping up presents for her friends and cousins. She becomes extra helpful in the weeks leading up to Christmas to try to get Jeff and me to buy her that special present she wanted. She gets so excited on Christmas Eve that she cannot get to sleep. She gets up extra early on Christmas day to open her presents.

Being able to play a musical instrument has always been my ambition. I encourage Emma to learn the piano. She is quite good but not a natural. It is probably because there is no one particularly musical in my or Jeff's family. I also encourage Emma to learn some Chinese, just sufficient to have a simple conversation with my parents or write a few words.

Emma takes after Jeff at sports, she is good at swimming and running. Jeff and Emma enjoy watching sports together. She knows all about the off-side rule and can name all the players in the premier division. Jeff encourages Emma to take part in a fun run with him. Taking part in sports helps her to build confidence, learn about team work, experience the joy of winning and the disappointment of losing.

At weekends and school holidays, we take Emma to visit museums, farms, theme parks and other places of interest. Emma loves animals. She enjoys her visits to the London Zoo, London Aquarium, Natural History Museum, Godstone farm. She loves going to theme parks such as Thorpe Park and World of Chessington and of course Disneyland. Since we are members of the National Trust, Jeff and I take her to visit NT properties to develop her interest in gardening and history. Emma enjoys her holidays abroad experiencing different climates, languages, food and culture.

Even though we live a long way from Jeff's parents, Emma has a particular close relationship with her grandmother. Emma just loves being with her grandmother who dotes on her – maybe it is because all her other grandchildren are grown up. She loved following her into the kitchen and watching her cooking. She follows her to the garden to feed the birds, sitting on her lap watching TV together, listening to her sing. Sadly Grandmother died when Emma was five years old. Emma is very upset at losing her grandmother.

Emma also loves to visit my parents. She is spoilt by my father who has a soft spot for her – she is allowed to stay up late and eat as much as she wants. Emma loves my mother's cooking. She enjoys playing with her cousins Christopher, Rebecca and Michelle. Being the oldest, she becomes the leader of the gang, leading them to mischief. She spends hours playing Gameboy with Christopher who is a Gameboy addict, drawing pictures with Michelle who is fond of drawing, or talking to Rebecca who is a chatterbox.

At school, Emma is good at mathematics and science subjects, but not so good at art and languages. She is a conscientious pupil, always handing in her work on time. She is not an extrovert, but she is sociable and she gets on well with teachers and fellow pupils. At home, she is a cheeky girl who knows how to get her own way, especially with Jeff. We do our best for her without spoiling her. We make sure she has good manners, keeps her room tidy and helps out with simple household chores.

When Emma reached puberty, the dreams faded out. I had expected arguments over what she could or could not wear, make up, jewellery, clothes, body piercing, hair colour and style, over who she made friends with, what places she could go to, how much time she could spend on the phone and what time she was expected home after a night out. Such dreams didn't materialise because they would have been too far from the reality. But the dreams I have described remain with me. They are just as real as the everyday Emma, they are somehow as much as Emma.

One day this sort of dream may come true, which is why the Rett Syndrome Foundation is spearheading the Research to Reality campaign to raise the much needed funding for finding a cure. See Appendix A for the latest work on this.

Chapter 8

Years of Normality

The possibility of stepping into a higher plane is quite real for everyone.
It requires no force or effort or sacrifice. It involves little more than changing our ideas about what is normal.
Deepak Chopra – Doctor, mind, body spirit author

This chapter covers the period between April 1998 and the end of 2006. It was a period of normality when we got on with daily life; no more endless hospital appointments, tests, treatments, sleepless nights. After our return from China, I decided it was more important to have a normal life than to keep trying for a miracle cure. I wanted to rediscover the joy of living, spend time with friends and family, go on holidays and learn new things.

Emma went willingly back to school following her stay in China. She did, however, miss her teacher Elaine who left when we were away. In September 1998, Emma was given a place at a local special school for children with severe learning difficulties. The school has wide expertise in special needs and they also have experience in teaching children with RS. Another Rett girl Sara had attended the school before Emma. Some of the teachers had learned a lot about RS from teaching Sara. One of them, Alison, was close to Sara and her family. Alison was also the first secretary of the Rett Syndrome Association in the UK when it was founded in 1985.

Jeff and I are pleased with the education and support Emma receives from school. Emma really thrives on the attention she had from the staff and the friendship from the other children. As she has grown older, her eye contact and concentration has improved. It is lovely to see Emma smile when I speak to her or sing to her. She has also developed a new interest in books – she enjoys being read to and she loves looking at the pictures. She also enjoys walking. She likes to look at the flowers in people's gardens and listen to birds sing. I settled in quickly after my return from China. While we were away Jeff had started piano lessons. I had always wanted to play the piano but my parents could not afford the lessons. It was wonderful to have an opportunity to learn and Albert the tutor was happy to take me on. So there I was, starting to learn to play the piano aged nearly forty. This was not only a pleasure for me, it was also a way of connecting with Emma. Through music, I can communicate with her. It is wonderful to see her smile when I play a tune that she recognises.

My desire to understand Emma and improve my

communication with her inspired me to take up an Open University course in Child Development in 1999. The course helped me to understand Emma's needs for love, attention and praise, and appreciate the importance of her having social interaction with other people. The year 1999 was a good year. Emma was happy at school, Jeff and I were happy at work. I also had more time for family and friends. For the first time since I had noticed something wrong with Emma, I felt there was some normality in my life. I felt so good that I decided to have a big party to celebrate my 40th birthday. Jeff had a marquee set up at the back of the house and about 30 neighbours and friends came to the party.

The year 2000 started well. We went to London to see the Millennium celebration in Pall Mall and Jubilee Gardens with Emma, Jeff's brother and sister-in-law. We were full of optimism for the new millennium. As I was driving into work one day, I heard on my car radio that the bank I worked for had been taken over by a larger bank. At ten o'clock, we were told that it was a merger and not a takeover. There was no immediate plan to close branches or call centres, or to merge support services such as accountancy and IT. Changes would be gradual, and any redundancies would be made on a voluntary basis.

2001 was a big year for Emma. We went to Australia to attend my sister Mary's wedding reception. We thoroughly enjoyed our holiday. The most memorable part was the drive along the Great Ocean Road and visiting the towns and villages en route. There is so much open space and so much natural beauty. It was also wonderful to enjoy the warm Australian welcome from my sister Mary's friends and the hospitality from her new husband David's family. Jeff and I had two days on our own in Sydney. I was pleased to be able to enjoy the beautiful scenery together with Jeff. We took the opportunity to have a three-week holiday in Hong Kong, Melbourne, Sydney and Singapore. It was a wonderful holiday. We met up with relatives and friends in the different countries and enjoyed visiting places. The highlights for Emma were the Ocean Park in Hong Kong, the Melbourne Aquarium and Melbourne Zoo, and the Bird Park in Singapore.

Emma's tenth birthday in December of that year brought both sadness and joy. Jeff and I decided to have a party to mark her milestone birthday. November was a manic month trying to get things organised. I was inundated with phone calls. Joan, our neighbour, who was making a cake, wanted to know what decoration to put on it, My friend Grace helped me with the catering. She wanted to know what food I wanted for the party. Other parents wanted to know what Emma would like for her birthday present. I really wished I knew what Emma wanted. All these questions brought home to me my inability to communicate with Emma. Despite not being able to make any decisions about what she wanted for her party, Emma greatly enjoyed seeing her friends, eating lots of food and being the centre of attention.

Jeff wrote a travel log for Emma during our visit to Australia. I thought it was a brilliant idea. Although Emma enjoyed the visit I was not sure if she could remember any of it. If there should be a cure for Emma one day, she would have no memory of her past. It would be such a tragedy. With her tenth birthday coming, I thought it was important to make a record of our experience. The result was 'Getting to Know Emma', a book I finished in 2002. Jeff helped me to produce 200 copies and we managed to sell them through the internet. Most of the copies were sold to people in the UK. We managed to sell a few copies in the USA with help from Emma's headmaster. Even though I could not get the book published properly it was a cathartic experience for Jeff and me. It was also encouraging to learn that people who read it found it comforting. We have received a lot of feedback, mainly from families with disabled children, some from teachers and nurses who work with children.

In 2003, Emma was allocated a place at the local respite care centre allowing her to stay in the centre for two nights a month. This was wonderful for Jeff and me and also for Emma. It gave us the freedom to go out to see a film or go to a restaurant on our own. It helped Emma to become more independent and learn to share things with other children. At home, she has exclusive use of the television. In the centre, she has to share with other children and watch programmes that she may not like.

In that year, 88 of my colleagues were made redundant. Although it was voluntary, the alternative of not taking redundancy was to relocate more than 200 miles away. This was very unsettling for us. People tried to avoid being made redundant by moving to important or strategic projects or to go to evening classes to train for an alternative career outside the company. A big change came in 2004 when my employer decided to outsource the IT work to an IT facility management company.

This meant that we would be working for the IT company rather than the bank. This completely changed the way we worked. The IT company has large off-shore centres that provide helpdesk and IT development facilities. We could no longer work with our clients directly. All our clients' requests for new work or help to solve problems had to come through our service desk. Our access to the data was limited which made it difficult to do our work. The hardest thing to get used to was the company's culture – instead of encouraging staff to work together as a team, we were made to compete with each other. Although my colleagues and I tried not to be influenced by this ethic, we knew we must not get on the wrong end of the performance curve.

Becoming a teenager was not easy for Emma nor for us. Emma went through the hormonal changes of a normal teenager but her inability to express her feelings made life very frustrating for her. She hates being put to bed at half-past eight. Most nights she just cries until she wears herself out. She has also become fussy about food. She does not like having leftovers from the previous day or meals without meat. She moans and groans when she becomes bored. This is particularly difficult during winter months when we cannot go out due to bad weather.

Emma's physical growth is also causing us problems. She has become too big for us to get her up and down the stairs. We had to get a stair lift fitted and a bath lifter to get her in and out of the bath. Her growth has accelerated the scoliosis (bend in her spine). She has to wear a jacket made of plaster to slow down the development of the curvature. The jacket is very uncomfortable and is a source of irritation for Emma, especially at mealtimes.

Her behaviour and size limit our choice of holidays. We find it difficult to travel with Emma by air. In the last four years, we have taken our holidays in France or in England. We have to choose our accommodation carefully; we can only choose single storey buildings because we cannot get Emma up and down stairs without a stair lift. Getting her in and out of the bath is always a problem but we have been managing so far. We need to read up about the resort carefully to avoid getting ourselves into difficulties on cobbled streets or lots of steps.

Let us catch up with Jeff here. He missed Emma and me very much when we were in China. He was pleased when we came back. Although things were difficult with both of us working full time, we managed with the help of our childminder Vicky. In November 1998, Jeff turned 50. It was a financial milestone for Jeff; it enabled him to start drawing his company pension and to take a lump sum to pay off the mortgage. We celebrated with a holiday in Euro Disney.

When Jeff's IT contract ended in early 2000, he was offered a permanent job in the development team doing work to replace an old computer system. He did not enjoy this work because it was mundane. Suddenly, a few months into his new work, he decided to resign after a disagreement with his manager. He did not consult me and I was quite shocked.

Jeff has an income from his pension and there was no pressure for him to find another job, so he decided to take early retirement and do as he pleased. In some ways, it made things easier for me as I did not have to worry about Emma's care during school holidays and when she is unwell. I thought it would be a good idea for Jeff to have a part-time job to bring in some income and to have something to keep him occupied. I felt, however, that he had not considered what effect this sudden change to house husband would have on our relationship.

The situation improved slightly when he acquired an allotment and started doing an Open University course. 2001 was a busy year for him: he organised our holiday in Australia, supervised work on the conservatory, and did most of the organisation for Emma's 10th birthday party. He enjoyed the holiday in Australia very much. It was the first time he had visited the country. We had a conservatory built in the spring and Jeff was at home to ensure that the work was carried out properly.

Jeff's father's health deteriorated rapidly in 2002 and he was diagnosed as suffering from dementia. Jeff went to visit him in Warwick regularly. His father was found wandering in the street at night. He came and stayed with us for a week but it was more difficult for him in a house he was not familiar with. Jeff's sister became the main carer, visiting nearly every day and his neighbours kept an eye on him. We managed to find a suitable care home but his condition deteriorated rapidly. Towards the end of his life, he was unable to recognise me or his grandchildren, and he confused Jeff with his brother and his daughter Carol with his wife. It must have been heart- breaking for Jeff to see his father suffering. Jeff's father died of pneumonia in 2003. All the surviving members of his army regiment came to his funeral dressed in uniform, some in wheelchairs and some with walking sticks. I was so moved to see them that I burst into tears.

When Jeff completed his Open University course in 2004, he began to get bored and became more reclusive. I tried to persuade him to do some voluntary work, but the only thing that I managed to persuade Jeff to do was to help out at Emma's school twice a week during lunch hours. He enjoyed being at the school and he was good with the children. He later got involved in building a sensory garden for the school. It took months of hard work from my colleagues at the bank through the community work scheme, parents and staff from Emma's school to complete the project. Jeff played an important part in the project and he was pleased with the result.

After that, he seemed to run out of things to do so he took up buying and selling on Ebay as a new hobby. He spent a lot of time on the computer. He became less and less communicative. He also became less willing to go out. We used to make an effort to go out in the evenings when Emma was at respite. Increasingly, Jeff just bought DVDs to watch at home.

Things became extremely difficult for me in 2005 and 2006. Emma's teenage tantrums made me feel helpless. I did not know what to do to stop her crying at night because she did not want to go to bed. I found it difficult when she burst into tears in the supermarket or shopping centre. I found it more difficult when people started staring at her or when children teased her and called her a big crying baby. I am sure this affected Jeff too, but he would not talk to me about it. Work became more and more stressful. With more people being made redundant, I had to take on more work and learn more new skills. Some days when I left work, I could not remember what day of the week it was, whether I had had any lunch or where I had parked my car. The sad thing was that home was no longer my sanctuary. There was nowhere for me to go for peace and refuge. Sometimes when I was stuck in traffic coming home from work, I had this mad idea of taking a different turn, disappearing and taking on a different name and a new life.

The title 'Years of Normality' may seem inappropriate for this chapter because there were sad and difficult events during these years; things such as Jeff's father passing away, Emma's teenage tantrums, Jeff becoming more isolated, my work problems, and my deteriorating relationship with Jeff. But for me, normality means stability and routine. During these years, I lived in the same house, worked in the same office,

Emma was in the same school. This may seem banality to some people, but to someone like me who had been to six different schools and has lived in many different places, it means normality.

These years of normality were important to me. The stability enabled me to recover from the trauma of Emma's diagnosis, gave me time to establish good relationships with friends and neighbours, build up financial security and strength to cope with the stormy weather ahead.

Part 2

In the Field of Battle

Chapter 9

A New Patient

We are not ourselves. When nature, being oppressed, commands the mind to suffer with the body.
William Shakespeare

Most people remember 1987 for the two tumultuous events of the Great Storm and Black Monday. But it was a special year for me – Jeff and I got married in September and I started a new job in a medium-sized bank in December. Both my marriage and my work have gone through troubled times in recent years. I was hoping 2007 would be a year for me to turn both around because it was going to be the Year of the Pig – a good year for me according to the Chinese horoscope. It turned out to be a stormy year for my relationship with Jeff and at work. It all began on an ordinary Monday morning.

Monday 29/01/07
Jeff woke up with a sore throat, feeling lighted-headed and dizzy. He said that he thought it was throat cancer. I was taken aback by this comment. It was unlike Jeff to make such

an irrational statement. He said he was going to see the doctor the next day but I could see he needed to see the doctor sooner. I rang the surgery and the receptionist told me all the doctors were busy and they could not fit him in. I insisted he must see a doctor because he was suffering from a lot of pain. Jeff was seen by a locum at noon but no medication was given to him. He was just told to take paracetamol.

Tuesday 30/01/07
Jeff took paracetamol as instructed by the doctor but there was no improvement. He was getting more convinced that he was suffering from throat cancer. He became more withdrawn than usual, spending all evening in the computer room. Jeff normally sleeps well but that night he was tossing and turning.

Wednesday 31/01/07
At around 4 am, I was woken up by noises downstairs. I went down to the dining room and found Jeff laying out lots of papers on the dining table. When he saw me, he told me that he was going to die soon and he needed to hand over all the paperwork to me, so that I would know what to do when he was gone. I told him not to be ridiculous, he was only suffering from a sore throat and he would get better soon.

He would not listen to me. He made me sit down next to him and started going through the various bills and how to pay them and the different bank statements. Then he took me into the computer room, logged on to his internet account and showed me how to process the account and then his Ebay accounts.

I rang work to say that I needed to take a day off. After the school bus took Emma to school, I took Jeff to the A & E department at the local hospital. After waiting a few hours, Jeff was seen by a young doctor. After checking his throat, he could not find anything wrong, so he told Jeff to take Neurofen to stop the pain. Jeff was upset by the way the doctor spoke to him. He kept saying to me: He did not believe I was ill. He thought I was a malingerer.

Friday 02/02/07

Jeff phoned me at work, saying he had been to see the Chinese doctor in the town centre. He had been through a session of acupuncture, massage and cupping therapy (it involves placing heated cups over the skin to encourage blood flow and ease stress, aches and pains), and given some tablets. He had paid £1032 for a course of 24 treatment sessions. He had never experienced Chinese medicine before and had not believed much in it. I came home early because I was worried about him.

While we were in the kitchen cooking together, I asked him why he had spent so much money. He said it was because the GP and the A & E doctor had not listened to him and he wanted to have someone to talk to. At this point, he became very emotional and burst into tears. He told me that he was afraid of dying; he did not want to leave our daughter Emma and me behind. He was frightened to go to the other side and he had unfulfilled ambitions.

After I had put Emma to bed at nine, we had a chat about his throat. He was adamant that he had throat cancer. I thought it was just a throat infection. We discovered on the internet information about types of infection, bacterial and viral. The medicine he was given was for viral infection and I guessed it must be bacterial. Although the infection was not serious, the psychological impact it was having on Jeff was serious. I decided he must get seen to and get it cleared up even though it was 11 pm. I rang the emergency number and was told to take Jeff to the local hospital to see the emergency duty doctor. We got to the hospital just before midnight.

Saturday 03/02/07
We sat and waited until 1 am and Jeff was seen by a duty doctor. I was worried that Jeff would start telling the doctor that he had throat cancer and get sent away with more paracetamol, so I told the doctor what had happened.

The doctor found pus at the back of Jeff's throat and he diagnosed that it was caused by bacterial infection. He was given Amoxicillin and Co-codomal. I felt that he was given the correct diagnosis at last.

Even though the medication was reducing the symptoms, he became more and more irrational. He complained about the skin on his face burning and of a very sore throat. He got himself into strange positions to relieve pressure on his throat: for example, he tilted his head back and made a neck brace to hold his head up. He then thought his poor posture was causing dislocation of his neck and shoulders. He studied a book on the Alexander Technique and practised the exercises obsessively to correct his posture.

Sunday 04/02/07

When he woke up on Sunday, his face was less red and he looked better. But he was in an anxious state and said his neck was broken. I told him it was not possible. He would not be able to hold his neck up or to speak if his neck was broken. It was no use. I knew there was something very wrong with his mental state. I did not know what to do, so I decided to phone George, a family friend who is a psychiatric nurse living in Gloucester. I told him about Jeff's condition and he advised me that I should get him admitted to hospital. He kindly offered to help if I had difficulty getting Jeff admitted.

Jeff was also concerned that the medication was not working fast enough to relieve the symptoms. He tried to calm himself by curling his body into the foetal position. He stayed in that position for about ten minutes. When he stood up he became agitated and he hyperventilated. He had to be taken to A & E by ambulance. He told the doctor he had throat cancer and possibly kidney failure because he was urinating frequently. The doctor assured him it was not throat cancer or kidney failure but that did not stop him from worrying. He had a shower to calm himself down and he said his skin was peeling off in the shower. I had to make him stand in front of a mirror to convince him that his skin was not peeling off.

It was very late when Jeff went to sleep exhausted. Although I was exhausted, I could not sleep – I had a lot of thinking and planning to do. What was I to do with Emma? With Jeff becoming increasingly unstable, I needed to get Emma respite care or get someone to look after her in the evening. What was I to do about work? I decided I could not leave Jeff on his own, I needed to be home with him. So, at two in the morning I sent an email to my team leader to say Jeff was unwell and I needed to stay at home to look after him for a few days. What was I to do about Jeff? I really did not have any idea.

Monday 05/02/07

After Emma went to school. I tried to find all the help I needed. I rang up social services to get respite care. They did not have any vacancies, but they put Emma on the waiting list. I rang up our neighbour Joan to ask her to get Paul, the pastor in her church, to come and see Jeff.

All morning Jeff talked, mainly about the different illnesses he thought he was suffering from such as throat cancer, skin cancer and kidney failure. At lunch he said he was suffering from rigor mortis. I said you could only get rigor mortis when you were dead. Late afternoon, he told me he was going to die soon, then collapsed onto the floor. I had to go next door to get Len and Sandra to help. They tried to reason with him and it was impossible. Sandra could see Jeff was very anxious so she sat with him and showed him some breathing exercises to calm him down. After Sandra went home, Jeff and I had a long chat. In fact, it was Jeff who did most of the talking, which was unusual. He told me I was his best friend – something he had never told me before. He said that after he died he wanted me to marry again, but he wanted me to marry someone who would be willing to take on Emma. I told him he was not going to die but he made me promise that I would do as he asked.

Because of Jeff's recent interest in an afterlife I asked Pastor Paul to talk to Jeff as I was unable to answer his questions about the other side. They had a long chat in the conservatory. The talk seemed to calm him down. I did not know what they talked about. I guessed Jeff must have asked Paul a lot of questions about life after death.

After dinner, Jeff's sister Carol rang. Jeff told Carol that he had a sore throat and the medicine was not working and it was giving him some strange symptoms. Carol thought that Jeff might be allergic to Penicillin and should not be taking it. Afterwards, Jeff refused to take Amoxicillin because it contains Penicillin. Later on in the evening, he hyperventilated again and I had to call an ambulance. Before the ambulance came, he said he needed more air and ran out of the house. I had to run after him in my pyjamas with a paper bag. Using this has often helped him when hyperventilating. When the ambulance came, he told the two medics that his lungs had collapsed. The men were patient with Jeff. They showed him on the monitor that his lungs were functioning and that he just needed to breathe more slowly. The ambulance men left when Jeff managed to breathe normally without help.

After Jeff went to bed, I had to start making plans for the next day. I did not know how much poor Emma understood. All the noise must have been very upsetting and frightening for her. I thought I would ask Kim, a lady who works in Emma's school who occasionally baby-sits Emma to help the next evening. Also, I needed to find out what was wrong with Jeff.

Tuesday 06/02/07

I rang the doctors' surgery first thing in the morning and managed to get an appointment for the afternoon. I also rang Kim at school and she agreed to come that evening. By now, I was getting rather nervous being in the house alone with Jeff. I rang George and asked if he could come and stay with me because I was too frightened. George said he could come the next day after taking his father for a hospital appointment.

Sandra came over to see if there was anything she could do to help and I told her I was worried about driving Jeff in my car because I might panic if he started behaving strangely. Sandra offered to drive us to the surgery to see the doctor. The diagnosis was Somatisation (a neurotic disorder in which the patient believes that he is suffering from a serious illness). The doctor referred Jeff to a clinical psychiatrist but the appointment was for Friday. I did not know how to get through the day let alone get through to Friday. After we got home he became agitated. He had a problem with breathing and he said he needed more air and tried to put the vacuum cleaner pipe down his throat.

I had to get help from Len and Sandra. Shanti and Tamara

116

on the other side heard the commotion and also came over to help. We managed to stop him doing damage to himself. When Joyce and Reg from two doors down found out what had happened, they came to see us. They were concerned about Jeff, they phoned and asked their daughter Joanne who is a clinical psychologist what to do. Joanne said that we must get Jeff to see the duty psychiatrist in A & E and get an immediate referral.

In the evening he hyperventilated again. Paramedics came and did lots of tests to assure him there was nothing wrong with him. They spent over an hour with him to show him that he was not suffering from any of the conditions that he claimed he was suffering from. They told him to carry on taking Amoxicillin and to drink plenty of water. While this was going on, Emma was being looked after by Kim in another room. Shanti knew I was worried about Emma being frightened by Jeff's behaviour. She offered to have Emma in her spare bedroom. After Kim left, I changed Emma into her nightdress and took her to Shanti's house for the night.

When I returned to the house, I found Jeff taking large quantities of Amoxicillin and drinking too much water. I had to hide the Amoxicillin but I could not stop him drinking water incessantly. That night, I could not sleep in fear of Jeff finding the Amoxicillin. Around 11:30pm, Jeff dozed off, so I had a short nap. I was woken up by Jeff rummaging through the drawers in the kitchen. When I got to the kitchen, he was about to swallow the tablets he found. I snatched them from him and ran upstairs. He ran after me. He grabbed the collar of my blouse and dragged me towards him. He nearly choked me. He got hold of my hands and pried them open and took the tablets from me. He gulped them down in one go. He then went into the bathroom to drink water.

I did not know who to turn to at midnight. Out of desperation I rang my sister Mary in Australia. I told her what was happening to Jeff. Jeff agreed to talk to Mary because she is a psychiatric nurse. Mary told Jeff if he drank too much water the electrolytes (a "medical/scientific" term for salts, specifically ions) in his body would become over diluted and he would suffer from water intoxication which could cause death. Jeff said his throat was dry and sore, Mary suggested he suck an ice cube. This seemed to soothe Jeff's throat and he stopped drinking incessantly.

Wednesday 07/02/07
As soon as Jeff woke up, he started doing some very strange movements; going round in circles in an anti-clockwise direction. He said this would help him travel back in time to the point when he did not have throat cancer or kidney failure. He became agitated and hot and the exercise did not work. He tried to swallow an ice cube. He nearly choked himself. He put his finger down his throat to get the ice cube out and caused himself to vomit all over the carpet.

I went over to Shanti's house to bring Emma back and got her ready for school. After the school bus picked Emma up at around 8:45am, I took Jeff to A & E and asked to see the duty psychiatrist for an assessment. We waited for hours in the hospital. Jeff spent most of the time demanding water and making numerous trips to the toilet.

I had to follow him up and down. During one of the trips, I saw one of the paramedics who had come to help Jeff the previous night. He came over for a short chat. I told him I was still unable to get Jeff admitted to hospital. He was sympathetic – but said that for admission you need to prove he is a danger to himself or others.

A doctor saw Jeff at around 11 am but he was not the duty psychiatrist. He had a look at his throat and told him to carry on taking the medicine. He told us the psychiatrist was busy and we had to wait until the afternoon to see him. This wasn't possible until 3 pm. Emma was due to be back by 3:45pm. I rang up the school and asked the deputy headmaster to find someone to look after her.

We were eventually seen by the duty psychiatrist. He did an assessment on Jeff but concluded that Jeff did not need to be in a hospital. I explained that Jeff was in a very agitated state, but the psychiatrist said he could not prescribe any medication. He told me I could try another hospital a few miles away.

I took Jeff there. He was seen by a psychiatrist and a nurse. After more assessment and lots of pleading from me, he was given medication (Zopiclone and Diazepam) to calm him down and to help him to sleep.

When we got home it was nearly 8 pm. I was cold, tired and hungry and there were 27 messages on the answer machine. After going through all the messages, I found one from the deputy headmaster saying that Emma had been taken into emergency respite care. There was another message from Brenda, my childminder who had learned that Emma was at the respite care centre from her daughter Wendy who works there. Brenda said she was coming round at 9 pm to take Emma's things to the respite care centre for me. Just when I was about to get to the end of all the messages, there was a knock on the door. It was Shanti from next door with a big bowl of hot soup. Jeff and I were hungry and cold, the hot soup went down a treat. While Jeff settled down to watch television, I packed a bag with some clothes and toiletries for Emma. Brenda arrived promptly at nine to pick up Emma's bag. I gave her a quick update of what happened in the last few days and thanked her for her help.

George arrived not long after Brenda left. I was so relieved to see him. Jeff was pleased to see him too because he wanted to talk to someone with medical knowledge about his problems. Jeff had a good sleep that night with the help of the latest prescription and the relaxation technique he learned from George.

Thursday 08/02/07
I did not realise I had been completely cut off from the real world in the last few days. When I opened the curtains, the garden was covered in thick snow. I had not watched television nor read the newspaper for nearly a week. I had

another surprise when I opened the fridge door: I had run out of milk and I discovered the orange juice had gone off. I left George to care for Jeff and drove to the local supermarket to get some supplies.

Jeff poured out all his problems to George. He told George that he had a long-standing problem with a very hot head, bad posture and sore throat. He had not done anything about these and they were now becoming so serious that he was going to die, and it was all his fault. George listened patiently and tried to assure him that it was not his fault. Jeff dutifully carried out relaxation exercises as instructed by George. I took the opportunity to clean up the mess on the carpet and soiled clothes left by Jeff in the last few days. After dinner, Jeff watched some sports programme on television with George so I went into the conservatory to do some ironing. I then went into the kitchen to make a cup of tea. I noticed George was asleep on the sofa in the sitting room and there was no sign of Jeff. When I went into the kitchen I found a knife with blood on the kitchen floor. I screamed and ran upstairs to look for Jeff. George ran up after me.

We found Jeff sitting on the bed with blood running down his right leg. He told us that he had felt a lot of pressure on his leg and he had to cut it to relieve the pressure. George dialled 999 and called for an ambulance. In about 20 minutes, a police car and an ambulance arrived. Two policemen and two ambulance men came into the house. Jeff refused to go with the ambulance men. He told them he did not want to go to hospital because he wanted to die at home. The ambulance men told him that he needed to have treatment at the hospital. The policemen also tried to persuade him. Jeff eventually agreed to go but he wanted George to be in the ambulance with him. I followed the ambulance in my car to the hospital.

I thought Jeff would be admitted to a psychiatric ward straight away but we were taken to the A & E to wait for Jeff to be assessed. We arrived there around 9:40pm. Jeff was shouting loudly. The security guard walked up and down to make sure he was not causing anyone harm. I felt extremely embarrassed about Jeff's behaviour. After about 15 minutes, we were seen by the triage nurse (someone who assesses a patient's condition and determines that patient's priority for treatment) who took down Jeff's details. He told us the crisis team were finishing for the night and that he had to get a consultant from one of the psychiatric wards to assess Jeff. We were given a cubicle to sit in while we waited for Jeff to be seen.

It seemed like an eternity with Jeff going into the toilet numerous times to drink water or relieve himself. I had to follow him to make sure he did not disappear. At one point, he got fed up waiting and tried to run away. When George tried to stop him, he got angry and tried to attack George. Eventually a psychiatric nurse came to the A & E to take Jeff for his assessment. The consultant saw Jeff first. After 10 minutes, Jeff came out of the room to go to the toilet. When he walked past me to go back to the consultant, I noticed he had forgotten to do his zip up. I tried to tell Jeff, but George stopped me. He told me I should let the consultant see Jeff in that state. After Jeff had his assessment, I saw the consultant on my own. I told her about the chain of events leading to his self-harm incident. She told me that the assessment showed Jeff was suffering from psychosis and he needed treatment in the hospital. I was so relieved that he was to be admitted at last. Jeff willingly went up to the ward with the nurse. George and I went with him. Two nurses came to help him into his room.

He was fine until George and I were ready to leave. He wanted to leave with us and when one of the nurses tried to stop him he started kicking and screaming. The other nurse had to press the panic button. This triggered the alarm and turned on the flashing lights. Other nurses came in from the staff room to help to restrain Jeff. One nurse had to give Jeff an injection to tranquilise him. It was very sad, but I felt relieved that he was safe and he was getting the support he needed. When George and I left the hospital, it was nearly 1 am Friday 09/02/07.

Chapter 10

Finding Reinforcements

*What the world needs is a new kind of army –
the army of the kind.*
Cleveland Amory, Author.

Friday 09/02/07

George and I got back from the hospital about 1:30am. It had
been a hell of a day. I opened a bottle of red wine. We talked
and talked, mostly about how Jeff had got into such a state.
George explained to me that Jeff was suffering from severe
depression and it would take a while to recover. George is a
good listener, not only because he is a psychiatric nurse but
also because he is a carer to his brother and mother. It was
good therapy to talk after two weeks of chaos, panic and
anguish. During the past week, I had slept very little and I
was exhausted. When I finally got to bed about 3 am, I fell
asleep straight away.

In the morning, my whole body was shaking. I had a long hot
bath and that helped to calm me down. I weighed myself and
found that I had lost 5 lb. I must have burnt off a lot of energy
since Jeff became ill. I felt empty physically and emotionally.

George woke up around 10 am. I told him about the shaking and he said that was post-traumatic stress. He advised me to see my GP as soon as possible to get some medication. Later on, George helped to draw up a list of things to take to Jeff. I rang the hospital to find out how Jeff was. The duty nurse told me Jeff had refused to take medication and had needed to be tranquillised by injection. She told me I could visit in the afternoon.

George went to stay with our mutual friend Peter. It was strange to be on my own. The house was in a mess and I spent the day cleaning. I had not seen Emma since Wednesday morning. I decided to see Emma first to put me in a positive mood before visiting Jeff. Emma was happy at the respite care home, but she looked confused to see me. The staff there told me she had been a little weepy at times, but on the whole she was fine. I was not sure if Emma understood what had happened.

Jeff was in a secure ward. I had to sign in at the reception and then wait outside a locked door for someone to let me in. A nurse came to open the door and took me to see Jeff. On the way to his room, the nurse told me that he was agitated. He had been knocking on other patients' doors. He drank water incessantly and had to be changed about five times. He was lying on the bed heavily sedated, wearing a green hospital gown, unshaved, hair uncombed. He recognised me, but he was still talking nonsense about kidney failure and drinking a lot of water to flush out his system. I told him that I had been to see Emma at the respite care home. I then asked him who Emma was. Jeff said she was my daughter. The visit ended on a positive note. Just when I was leaving Jeff said that he was winning a slow battle.

Saturday 10/02/07

I could not bear to be in the house on my own. I had to get out. I met up with my sister Jane in London. We had lunch and I told her all the things that had happened. Jane found it incredible because Jeff had been such a calm person. I told her Jeff would be in hospital for a while and I needed someone to help me to look after Emma. Jane agreed to come and help. Later, we went to see the musical Guys and Dolls. I had great difficulty concentrating. On my way home, at Victoria Station, I had a panic attack – I felt hot and sick, my heart was beating fast and sweat poured down my forehead. It took a few minutes to recover.

When I went to see Jeff that evening, he was more alert but still agitated. He did not want to stay in his room and he went for a walk. I followed him to the corridor. It was an eerie sight. There were a few other patients pacing up and down the corridor with blank looks on their faces – for a moment I thought I was on the film set of One Flew Over the Cuckoo's Nest. I had to follow him up and down in order to talk to him. When I asked the nurse to let me out, she told me to bring some shaving gel and a razor and some clothes for Jeff.

Sunday 11/02/07

I applied for another week's leave via email because it was

half-term for Emma. My team leader Ken told the head of the department about Jeff: they gave me time off as compassionate leave.

Emma's emergency respite care period was coming to an end on Monday and I needed to work out a rota of getting people to look after Emma when I visited Jeff. Brenda, our childminder, was brilliant. She increased the number of days she looked after Emma from two to four and she volunteered to pick Emma up from school. A friend Kathleen, and my sister Jane agreed to cover Friday and Saturday. I rang Kim, an assistant at Emma's school who sometimes babysits for us. Her husband told me she was in hospital. Even on her sickbed, Kim arranged for Evelyn, a friend and colleague, to look after Emma.

In the afternoon, I went to see the neighbours, Len and Sandra, Shanti and Tamara, Joyce and Reg, gave them an update on Jeff and thanked them for all the help they gave me. I wrote two letters to the school, one to the deputy headmaster to express my gratitude for his help and to Emma's form teacher explaining the situation at home and the new arrangement for Brenda to pick Emma up four days a week. Jeff was more coherent when I saw him. He said he was angry but did not know with whom, what or why. He also got attached to one of the nurses. He kept calling out for her to help him with things. He must have been exhausting to look after. I decided calming music was what he needed, so I brought him his MP3 player the next day.

Monday 12/02/07

I went to my GP. He was sympathetic about my problem. He had known me for over 15 years. He told me that I needed to have some tablets to help me to sleep. If I needed something stronger, then I should go back to see him. I felt it was a shame Jeff did not always see his own GP, who knew him well. GP's clinics do tend to be like assembly lines these days.

Jeff was a little better that day. He was able to concentrate for a little while. We sat down in the games area and played scrabble but, after about five minutes, Jeff lost his concentration and decided to take a walk. Then a young man came and sat down and talked to me. He thought I was a nurse and started telling me his life story. He was an intelligent young man and had ambitions to become a composer. He suffered from bipolar disorder and he was first admitted to hospital when he was only 18 during his first year at university. Since then he had been having relapses and had been in and out of hospitals.

This was the first time I had been mistaken for a nurse. As I discovered later, there were few permanent staff in the ward: most were agency nurses. Patients need stability and to see familiar faces. As I became a frequent visitor in the next few weeks, I had more and more people coming to talk to me. By the time Jeff left, I got to know nearly all the patients in the ward.

After visiting Jeff, I picked Emma up from Brenda's house. Not only was she a good childminder, she was knowledgeable on social services. Her daughter Wendy had just started working in the respite care home where Emma attends. During the past week of chaos, she had helped to organise Emma's life for me. Emma was pleased to be home where she could watch anything she liked on TV. She must have been missing Jeff, but she could not tell me. I was pleased to have her back. It had been strange being on my own for the last few days.

Tuesday 13/02/07

Emma returned to her routine of being picked up by the school bus. I told the driver Donna and escort Wendy about Jeff and the new arrangement of Emma being picked up by Brenda. They were flexible and did not mind the change.

Jeff wanted me to take him some books, clothes and other things, so I went through his bookcase and wardrobe. I found some clues to Jeff's depression. Jeff is normally tidy and I was surprised by the mess in his desk drawers – pens that did not work, paper clips and obsolete floppy disks everywhere. His clothes revealed more about his mental state – trousers with missing buttons, zips that do not work, split seams and frayed hems. Some of his shirts had stains. I also noticed the freezer was nearly empty.

Jeff had stopped going to the superstore recently and had opted to buy a little at a time from local shops. Jeff seemed happier when I visited him. He had found a new friend in a young Polish man. He taught Jeff to do Tai Chi and that seemed to calm him down. While they were practising Tai

Chi, a cheerful young man spoke to me in Cantonese. I found it difficult to believe there was anything wrong with him.

Wednesday 14/02/07
It was quite rare for me to have time at home. There were a lot of things that needed to be done in the house and in the garden, but I had not been able to get Jeff to do it or to get Jeff to pay someone to do it. I decided to have it all done while he was in hospital. I found someone to clean the drive and two men to repave the garden paths and steps and cut back the overgrown shrubs in the next few days.

Thursday 15/02/07
Things started to improve with Jeff. He stopped talking about illnesses and accepted that he was suffering from severe depression and needed help. He had got to know the staff better and had become friendly with other patients. His concentration was also getting better and he was able to do a mini-Sudoku and complete part of a crossword puzzle and do his Latin coursework. He also started to miss Emma and asked me how she was getting on. I later found out from the nurses that Jeff had been talking to them about her.

Friday 16/02/07
Joan had dinner with Emma and me that evening. While we were chatting after dinner, there was a knock on the door and I opened it to meet a girl who delivered a massive bouquet of flowers and a card from my colleagues. When I read the messages on the card, I burst into tears. For the last two weeks, I had tried to hold back the tears and had just got on

with what I had to do. Joan had known me since we moved to the house and shared our ups and downs and she told me it was good to cry. She was right.

Saturday 17/02/07

The following week, Emma went back to school and I decided to go back to work. I had worked out a schedule that I would work from 9:30am to 3:00pm in the office and then make up the hours in the evening or weekend working at home on my laptop. In order to work, look after Emma and visit Jeff, I needed to be organised. I had to resort to using a spreadsheet to plan my life. It was a sad thing to do but it was effective. The weekend was mostly spent on getting ready to go back to work and organising help for Emma.

Monday 19/02/07

Things went smoothly and according to plan. I managed to get Emma ready for school on time and I arrived at and left the office on time. Help with Emma was available when I needed it. It was hard work having to look after Emma, do the housework and fit in all the other things as well. Most nights I did not go to bed until twelve. Jeff was getting better slowly but steadily.

Friday 23/02/07

Nearly a whole week had passed without major problems and I was getting pleased with myself. At lunchtime, a nurse from the hospital rang me at work to tell me that they were going to let Jeff go home for the whole weekend. I could not believe that they had decided this without consulting me. So

I told the nurse that Jeff might be ready to come home but I was not ready to have him home. I told her about Jeff's incidents of harming himself and now I had Emma at home with me. I was not sure that Jeff would be able to cope with the stress. I told her I was prepared to have Jeff home for the day but not overnight. She went to consult the doctor and then agreed that Jeff would come home for the day on Sunday.

When I saw Jeff later that day, I explained to him why I was not ready for him to stay for the whole weekend. He was disappointed but he accepted that it was difficult for me to have him staying at night. I had to admit that I was apprehensive about being in a car with him and not knowing how he would react when Emma cried. We went home by taxi so that I could sit with him. We also decided that if there was anything that upset him, he would go into the computer room and put his MP3 on.

Sunday 25/02/07
Jeff greatly enjoyed his home visit. It was the first time he had seen Emma in over two weeks. He logged onto his computer, checked his email and played his favourite music. We had a big lunch and we went out for a walk afterwards. Jeff was very sad. Then it was time for him to leave. I went back to the hospital with him in a taxi.

Tuesday 27/02/07
The following week, Jeff had improved so much that he was allowed to go out with me to the hospital restaurant or have

a walk outside. His concentration was much improved and I discovered that the reason the doctor thought he was ready to come home for the weekend was that he had managed to complete a Sudoku and a crossword puzzle. I didn't agree with this assessment. My view is that intelligence and power of concentration have nothing to do with mental stability. I made this point clear in a letter I wrote to the consultant and ward manager and I asked to be consulted in advance if they wanted to let Jeff home next time.

Friday 23/03/07

Over the weeks, Jeff had continued to improve, had come home a few times, had stayed overnight and I felt more confident about him. Taking him in the car had been nerve-wracking though and I had insisted on his sitting still in the back. I made sure the doors were locked. I could not forget the occasion when on one journey to the hospital, he had threatened to jump out.

At the hospital, things were not easy. His Polish friend was moved to another ward and a few days later, Jeff was moved to a geriatric ward for a few days because of the shortage of rooms in his ward. He became increasingly bored and restless but, fortunately, was well enough to leave the hospital on the 23rd. I was pleased that he had made such good progress, but his coming home created a new set of challenges for me.

Chapter 11

Facing New Ordeals

It is impossible to win the race unless you venture to run, impossible to win the victory unless you dare to battle.
Richard M Devos, American tycoon

I was worried that Jeff would not be able to cope on his own at home, so I got permission to work at home for a while. Having the laptop and telephone conference facility enabled me to do most there.

Jeff seemed to be coping well. He took his medication without prompting and was able to do simple tasks in the house, but the anti-depressant and anti-psychotic drugs were making him very tired. He spent a lot of time at home sleeping. His Care Co-ordinator from the local Community Mental Health Team was fairly helpful. She found a Yoga class and a Tai Chi class for Jeff to attend and also persuaded Jeff to do a Latin course with the University of The Third Age. This was a useful addition to Jeff's course at the Open University. Paul, the local Pastor, came to visit regularly and Jeff got on so well with him that he was persuaded to go to church.

As described in chapter 9, Jeff had spent over £1,000 in a local Chinese medicine shop on 2nd February. I phoned the shop and the receptionist told me that I was too late because I had not asked for the money back within 28 days. I told her that I had asked for the money back the next day but she refused to acknowledge it and when I persisted the receptionist referred me to the head office.

I wrote to the sales manager several times and I had to obtain a letter from the doctors to prove Jeff was mentally unstable. I told the sales manager I was determined to get the money back even if I had to get the CCTV footage from the council to prove that I had been to the shop the day after or if I had to ask my neighbour to be a witness. I told them I was willing to go to court and that if I did not succeed, I would write to the local newspaper. They gave in eventually and I got a refund in May. I later learned from other carers that this is a common problem they have to deal with.

As Jeff regained more confidence and became less dependent on me, I felt able to go back to work full time in the office in June. Work had been enjoyable and it had provided a relief from the troubles at home, but recent changes had created a lot of stress.

Things were going well for Jeff for a while after he left hospital. He was, however, putting on a lot of weight because the anti-psychotic drug Olanzapine increased his appetite. His lethargy worried me. I tried to appear strong, but inside I was fragile. Then I remembered a leaflet about support for carers that I picked up from the psychiatric ward. I rang the number and I spoke to the Carers Support Worker, Helen from the NHS Trust. A few days later, Helen came to see me. She told me that I could ask Jeff's Care Co-ordinator to get a better understanding of his condition and medication. She gave me some information on MIND, on a 'Making Life Better' training course for carers and on a local charity for carers. I felt empowered after the meeting. For the first time, I felt able to do something positive to help Jeff instead of just fire fighting – I realised that there was special help available for carers.

I took Helen's advice to speak to Jeff's care co-ordinator and she suggested that we use the Family Consultation Service in the Community Mental Health Centre. The NHS Trust funds courses for carers on how to cope with the stress of caring and how to develop a positive outlook. The course, facilitated by a Relate counsellor, was based on elements of counselling and Cognitive Behaviour Therapy. Jeff went on the course and found it useful: He was able to cope better with Emma's teenage tantrums – crying at bedtime and sulking when she does not get the food or DVD she wants.

Jeff's care co-ordinator also arranged a family consultation for us. We talked to a team of three people: Two psychiatric nurses and one psychologist, while in another room there were two observers. We were encouraged to talk about our problems. Jeff was not forthcoming, but we got an idea of how burdensome it was for him to look after Emma. Deciding on our roles was difficult. Because I worked full time, Jeff was expected to do chores that he did not like to do and he felt it was my job to do the cleaning and ironing. I did not have the time and I was too tired after work to do these chores. I was happy to pay for someone to do it, but Jeff did not think it was necessary. After a few sessions, I therefore decided to bring the family consultation to an end.

I also contacted the local carers' charity to see if there were any services that I could use. Susan, on the helpline, was calm, understanding and reassuring and I decided to become a member so that I could receive the newsletter and I benefit from their stress-busting treatments. I decided to try their craniosacral therapy because I have a lot of problems with neck, shoulder and wrist pains through prolonged excessive use of computers.

The first session with Julie, the therapist, was most embarrassing. I burst into tears in front of this poor woman whom I had never met and I just cried uncontrollably. I guessed all these months of stress, coping with Jeff's mental illness, the demand of looking after Emma, the frustration at work, and the pressure of putting on a brave face was too much to bear and I had to let it out. Fortunately, Julie coped brilliantly with my problems. I was energised and ready to fight more battles.

There were more uncertainties at work. Our office building had been sold and we had to move to another location, not knowing when and where. The redundancy process was unpredictable and the appraisal system added more pain.

Most people in our office were given a poor rating for their performance. Some even had to go on the humiliating Performance Improvement Programme. The sickness level was high. Some people could not wait for the redundancy and decided to leave. Those left in the office were struggling to cope with the stress and workload.

One day, a colleague was distressed by the assessment of his work by the team that authorises changes to the computer system. I felt I had to speak up. I told them what I thought of the process. I did not want to see any of my colleagues ending up in a psychiatric ward. Everyone was surprised at my outburst. After the meeting, the manager asked to see me. He was worried about me not being myself and thought that I might still be suffering from post traumatic stress. I told him I was perfectly fine and I was being myself – my post traumatic stress just gave me the courage to speak up. I knew things would get even tougher in the months to come, but I was determined to stay until I got the redundancy payout.

We had a performance-related pay and bonus scheme. We had to be assessed every six months and our work had to be compared with colleagues in different parts of the country who were working on different projects. The review method tended to be based on the size of project and the number of people the person is in charge of rather than the level of expertise required to do the work and the amount of effort put into it. I was given a 'Below Average' rating in the last performance review. In fact, three out of six people in my team received 'Below Average' rating. I had always had an above average rating in my 19 years with the company. I suspect the rating had more to do with me coming to the end of my usefulness rather than with my performance. I was very angry. I had put in so much effort over the past few years that I had not immediately noticed that my husband was suffering from depression. I was now concerned to protect myself against constructive dismissal.

Normally, people were not willing to talk about their performance rating, especially when it is average or below. When other colleagues in the office heard about me raising a grievance, a number of them came to see me. They told me how angry they felt about the unfairness of the process and they were happy for me to use their cases to backup my own. It was encouraging to know that my colleagues were so supportive. The appeal process was protracted and more painful than the performance review process. I had to put into writing why I was not happy and I had to attend an interview. I spent a lot of time and effort into putting my case together, using the evidence of colleagues in the team but I was not allowed to use this. My appeal was not successful. I could have taken it to the next stage but I found that it would have created a lot of extra work and stress for my team leader Ken so I decided not to pursue my case.

Colleagues continued to talk to me about their work problems. Suddenly I became the agony aunt of the office. I had to do something about it. I identified a number of areas that needed improvement and produced a report: Two of my suggestions were adopted. The change review meeting format was improved and people working at night were given the taxi fare or the option to stay in a local hotel.

After months of waiting and speculation, finally in mid-August 2007 I was informed that my voluntary redundancy application was successful. My leaving date was to be at the end of November – two weeks short of my 20th anniversary with the company. I was able to make another 20th anniversary in September, my wedding anniversary. Our marriage had survived Emma's disability, the reversal of our roles and Jeff's mental illness. We decided to go to Edinburgh for a long weekend to celebrate.

Two weeks before that I emailed Professor Adrian Bird of Edinburgh University who has discovered that some of the symptoms of Rett Syndrome could be reversed. Professor Bird's secretary replied and arranged a meeting for us to see him in his office.

We had a wonderful time in Edinburgh. It was the first time since Jeff's breakdown that I felt I could relax, and forget the problems at home and at work for a few days. Being in Edinburgh gave Jeff newfound energy. We did a lot of sightseeing and swimming in the hotel pool. The meeting with Professor Bird gave us a big boost in morale. He explained his research to us and we felt encouraged that there was hope for Emma in the future. We came home on a high. Meanwhile, Jeff had decided he did not need his medication. October was a busy month for me. Before I left the company, I had to document all the systems I had worked on and to train two colleagues from overseas who were coming to stay in the UK for two weeks. The whole team had been busy preparing for their visit, for work and leisure. Emma had been given a few days in the respite care centre, so I planned to visit my parents as I had not seen them for a long time. Jeff was busy preparing for his Open University Latin exam.

A few days before the exam, Jeff started to get nervous. It was unlike him to be nervous about examinations. He already had a degree from the Open University. One day, when I returned from work, Jeff told me he thought there was still something wrong with him: His kidneys were not working properly. I guessed he was not taking medication. The pressure of the examination, my plan to go away for the weekend and an appointment with the dentist were getting on top of him.

I rang the crisis team and was told to take him to the Community Mental Health clinic to see a doctor the next day. We waited a long time, and we were seen by a psychiatric nurse eventually, but told we had to go to the doctor in the psychiatric hospital to get medication. Jeff had to go there on his own because it was time to pick Emma up from the respite care centre.

I was annoyed with Jeff for not taking the medication, so I told him he had to take responsibility for his own actions. Jeff was then given a higher dose of Olanzapine because of his condition. After a week or so, the delusions gradually disappeared. Because of the higher dosage, he was more tired and eating more. I could not take time off to look after him as the overseas colleagues had arrived and I also wanted Jeff to learn to be less dependent on me. I hoped that when I finished work in a few weeks time, I would be able to do more to help him.

The end of November finally came. Nearly twenty years of enjoyable work and friendship in that company came to an end. Twenty-two of us left the company. Those left behind were to be made redundant over the following year. Some people started looking for work as soon as they learned about the redundancy. I decided to have a few months off to find a suitable college for Emma when she leaves school in the summer of 2011. I also needed to think about my future. I knew it would not be easy for me to find another IT job at my age. Besides, I would not be able to find one locally. For the first time in my life, I did not know what to do.

Winter is always a difficult time for Jeff because he cannot work on his allotment and the darkness depresses him. When I was working, we seldom had time to do things together so I looked forward to this. We joined a badminton class and we did a start up your own business course. I also did some voluntary work to help the Rett Syndrome Association to find a replacement computer system. I really enjoyed having time off after working for 25 years full time. There was plenty to do; meeting up with friends, ex-colleagues and talking to neighbours.

In January 2008, I went to see the alternative therapist,

Deena, at the local carers' centre to have a massage. We had a chat about my redundancy and Jeff. Deena told me that she worked in a club for disabled people every Thursday and they needed male volunteers in particular. I knew Jeff would not go on his own so I went with him. We helped to make tea and coffee in the morning and prepare lunch. In the afternoon there were organised activities such as bingo and painting. The other volunteers were friendly and we got on well with them. After a few weeks, Jeff was content to go on his own but he was still negative. He was always saying 'I can't do it' or 'I don't want to do it' which I found it extremely frustrating.

Also in January, I had a phone call from Linda who works for the local carers' charity. She told me she had found my name on the list of people who are willing to do a talk. She asked if I would give a talk to a group of social workers about my experience as a carer the following week. I agreed to do it because I had done a talk about caring for Emma to a group of work experience students at Emma's school. Also, in the last few months at work, I had given presentations to colleagues.

I talked about my experience as a carer for both Emma and Jeff to a group of 12 newly recruited social and health professionals. I thought the talk went well. I managed to tell my story without becoming too emotional and it was a good audience; interested, sympathetic and responsive. Even though they knew there were problems with the services for the disabled and mentally ill, they were surprised at how much trouble I had in getting Jeff admitted to hospital. I gave another talk in February. After the talk, Linda told me the charity had a vacancy for the post of a Carers Support Worker. The job was to provide support to carers who look after someone with mental illness and to help provide training for people who work with mentally ill patients.

I passed the interview and the work was interesting and rewarding. Although I did not have any professional qualifications in the health and social services, I did have a lot of experience as a carer and I had first hand experience in dealing with the care services. Also, I know that the skills I had gained from my previous job were relevant, such as PC skills, time-management skills and training and coaching skills.

The knowledge I gained from my new job proved to be useful for coping with Jeff's behaviour. I realised I had to be patient, not to push him but to encourage him and to help him to build confidence. After working in the disabled club for a few months, Jeff felt confident enough to volunteer for teaching IT for the local Age Concern office in the summer. There were no immediate plans to run the courses so Jeff had to wait. Then a friend told me that her husband needed some help with his work on the computer. I asked Jeff whether he was willing to help and he agreed. They got on so well together that they remain friends even though the computer work finished long ago.

Jeff managed well in the summer despite not doing well with the allotment. In October, Age Concern contacted Jeff to ask him to run a three week IT course for their clients. The course was popular and Jeff found it rewarding. Also in October, Jeff was discharged from the Community Mental Health Team because he was managing well without help from his Community Psychiatric Nurse. He was now under the care of his GP.

Jeff turned 60 in November. We had a party to celebrate. It was the first time Jeff had had a birthday party since I had known him. He invited people from his church. It was wonderful to see his friends in the house. With his freedom pass he travelled around the local towns and explored London. At Christmas, Jeff received cards and presents from people he had helped and I could see he was moved by people's friendship and appreciation.

But this renewed confidence created a new problem because he decided he no longer needed the medication, saying that no medical professional had told him that he had to continue taking medication. February 2009 was a difficult month. Although I already had plans for the half term holiday in mid-February I had not planned for the heavy snowfall and for Emma catching a cold. She had to be at home for nearly two weeks so I feared Jeff might suffer a relapse through not taking medication and the strain of looking after Emma. My worst fear was realised when Jeff told me he had a sore throat and a stiff neck and he needed to see his GP.

Jeff rang up the surgery and the GP told him to go to the local hospital to have a blood test, and then make an appointment when the blood test result was produced. I was extremely worried about this delay in seeing the doctor and I asked Jeff to phone the Community Mental Health Team but they told him to see his GP. There was nothing we could do but wait. Jeff was getting more and more anxious about his symptoms and I had to relive the nightmare of his breakdown all over again. Meanwhile, my worries increased and I had great difficulty sleeping. One morning, after spending hours tossing and turning, I got up at 6am in the middle of February to go for a run. I felt a strange sense of calm after the run. That night, after Emma had gone to bed, I showed Jeff the journal I had kept about his breakdown and how it had affected me, together with the notes that George had taken and the notes that he had written himself.

Jeff was shocked. He realised what he had put me through and promised that he would take the medication after seeing the doctor and that he would attend classes to help him manage his anxiety and learn about recovery. A few days later, Jeff and I went to see the GP who thought Jeff should have anti-depressants to contain his anxiety. I told the GP that the consultant at the Community Mental Health Centre had said it was the anti-psychotic drug that stopped his delusions but the GP checked the information about the anti-depressant and decided that was the more appropriate medication for Jeff. After taking the medication for three weeks, Jeff was getting worse. He started talking about suffering from different illness incessantly. It was difficult for me to deal with his delusional behaviour. It did not matter what I said, it would not make any difference.

It was especially difficult at the weekend when we were together a lot of the time with Jeff continually sounding off. On Sunday 24th February, after a sleepless Saturday night, I decided Jeff had to go into hospital, so I got up early in the morning, packed Jeff a bag, ordered a taxi and sent him off to the hospital where he had been admitted two years ago. Because of Jeff's previous record, Jeff was admitted straight away.

His second admission went a lot smoother than the first one in 2007. Some of the staff at the psychiatric ward still remembered him from the last admission and he was put on anti-psychotic drugs straightaway. There was now more help for carers, a room for family visitors and an information pack for carers.

However, I was still struggling, juggling caring with work. Jeff's admission coincided with work to be done to the gutter and the fascia board on the house. Everyday I had to get Emma ready for school, wait for workmen to come, go to work, come back at lunch time to check things were OK with the workmen, pick Emma up from Brenda, the childminder, cook dinner and do the housework. I managed to get through the three weeks while Jeff was in hospital with the help of my reliable army of my neighbour Joan, sister Jane, Emma's school assistant Kim and the indispensable Brenda. I was rather pleased with myself that I managed well without Jeff until I received an email from British Gas – the gas meter reading I submitted was far too high, I was asked to check the reading. I went into the garage to check – confident that I was right. Indeed, I had read it correctly, but I had read it from the wrong meter – the electricity meter.

Jeff was discharged from the ward after three weeks and he was put on a five week programme at the Day Treatment Clinic. The therapies there were effective. It was the ideal treatment for Jeff. He had to attend the clinic every day to see the doctors and the therapist and there were group therapies with other patients. He was able to be with Emma and me in the evening. I remained supportive, but deep inside I felt resentful and angry with Jeff for putting me through this hell again. I did not feel any sympathy for him. I felt this episode of psychosis was of his own doing. After many sleepless nights, I decided I should try counselling.

Counselling does not work for everyone and much depends on whether you find a counsellor that you get on with. I was fortunate. I was able to open up and discuss my problems with Jackie. I learned a lot from her, especially about asking for help, telling people the truth, managing difficult emotions such as anger and resentment, and looking after myself.

As time went on, things gradually settled back to normal. Jeff finished his therapy at the Day Treatment Centre, continued with his Art and Latin classes and with his voluntary work. He even found a friend in the Day Treatment Centre. After two months of counselling, my negative emotions were under control and I felt I was able to carry on my job as a carer.

Jeff's relapse is a typical pattern of recovery. Full of ups and downs. On the whole, Jeff is on the up at the time of writing. He is recovering well from his illness. He now recognises his problem with anxiety and he is willing to learn to control it. I just need to be patient and supportive, and keep fighting the battles.

In December 2009, Emma turned eighteen. She had a birthday party to celebrate her being an adult. It was a happy and a sad occasion for me. It was lovely seeing her and her friends enjoying the party, but sad that she cannot be independent and will lose touch with her school friends once she leaves school. Her back is affected by scoliosis and her joints have become more stiff, but we are grateful that she is still mobile. Apart from the occasional tantrum, Emma seems to be quite contented and generally happy. She is still able to go the respite centre and a Saturday Club for disabled children. We are determined to make the most of all the facilities available to Emma until she is nineteen.

I have come to the end of the more personal aspects of my story – my experience as mother and wife. It is time to talk about my work as a carers' support worker and trust carers' lead, and about the dedicated carers I have learned from.

Chapter 12

Sad, Mad or Bad

No stranger to trouble myself, I am learning to
care for the unhappy.
Virgil (70 – 19BC), The Aeneid

According to government statistics, one in four people suffer from mental illness at some stage of their lives. As some of the stories below testify, personal experience of mental illness can be useful for a carer.

We have seen our friend Darren helping Emma with the patterning exercise in 1995. He was gentle, introverted and highly intelligent; a promising young man. He had been a local chess champion when he was a teenager, won a place at Cambridge University, and became the European Shogi (Japanese chess) champion in his early twenties. He then suffered a breakdown and he stopped playing. Darren never gave us any reason for his breakdown. I gathered that he had never worked and needed medication for his depression. He developed an interest in music and he often met up with his friends to practise together. He also taught himself to read Chinese. In the years we knew him, Emma brought him out of his shell. He became less shy and more confident. He even brought along one of his friends to meet us.

When Darren's mother died after a short illness, he was forced to move out of the council house they shared. We helped him to move to a one-bedroomed flat, but it was too small for his possessions and we kept all his trophies in our garage. Darren got over the crisis with the support from his musician friends but he became withdrawn and his visits became less regular. I tried to keep in touch by phone and when I did not hear from him for a few weeks I went to his flat, got no answer and I pushed a note through his letter box and asked him to contact me. But I never heard from him again. A few days later, one of his friends contacted me to tell me Darren had died in a diabetic coma in October 1999 aged 46. Through his friend, I managed to get in touch with Darren's brother and gave him Darren's trophies.

Through my work as a Carer Support Worker, I often meet people with mental illness. One of the most inspirational people I have met through my work is Philip. I had to invite a speaker to talk about recovery for one of the courses I organised for carers. Someone in the office gave me his name. Philip came to my group and gave a very moving talk. Philip had been a schoolteacher with three children. He suffered a breakdown in his early thirties after his best friend died unexpectedly. He was diagnosed as having bipolar disorder.

During his long illness, which lasted 16 years, he had two acute episodes of delusions of grandeur. In the first he thought he was Jesus. In the second he thought he was the son of Hitler. His psychologist tried to convince him that he could not possibly be Hitler's son because he was born four years after Hitler's death. Philip found some way of justifying it to himself and others. He was admitted into a psychiatric ward seven times, his average stay being two to three months, some lasting six months. His illness took a toll on his family life, affecting his wife so badly that she also suffered from depression. The lowest point of Philip's life was when both his wife and he were admitted to the same ward, his three children had to be taken into care, he lost his job and his house, and was heavily in debt.

With a lot of determination, help from the health professionals, and support from family and friends, Philip managed to recover. He points out that people have different ways of coping with mental illness. He does not advise them to do what he does. He has a strict regime: good diet, plenty of exercise, takes medication and avoids stress. He goes into great lengths to avoid stress, arriving at least an hour before an appointment. He even stops watching television or listening to the radio to avoid hearing bad news. Out of hospital, he had difficulty getting a job so he did some voluntary work. Through that he obtained a job with the local Primary Care Trust to promote mental health awareness in schools, communities and businesses.

People who suffer from bipolar disorder used to be called manic depressives, experiencing extremely high (mania) and low (depression) moods. Mania can express itself in different forms such as restlessness, little need for sleep, racing thoughts, excessive euphoria and elevation of mood. The actor/writer Stephen Fry is bipolar. When he is in a manic stage, he is at his most creative and productive and when he is in a depressive stage, he feels unable to face the world. His documentary *The Secret Life of the Manic Depressive* for the BBC, broadcast in 2006 was enlightening.

James is a talented artist. I met him and his mother at an art exhibition. He went to art college when 18. After the first term at college he came home for Christmas. He told his mother that he had been cursed by an old lady who sat behind him on the coach. He had not secured his bag in the rack properly and it had fallen on her lap. His mother tried to assure him that he was not cursed and that the old lady had probably forgiven him. James would not listen to his mother.

James started telling people that he could hear voices saying unpleasant things to him. He became more and more withdrawn, would not go out and refused to take phone calls from his friends. He spent a lot of time in his room painting strange pictures. His mother tried to persuade him to see a doctor but James said there was nothing wrong with him. He could blame himself for some crime committed on television. His mother tried to reason with him saying he had been home all day and that he could not possibly have committed the crime. The following day, two policemen called and told her that someone in the house had confessed to killing a young boy.

Despite protests from James' mother, the policemen took James to the police station. There he was seen by a psychiatrist and diagnosed with schizophrenia and admitted to a psychiatric ward. After four months, he was discharged and went back to college. He was well until his final year when he began to experiment with drugs. On ketamine, he imagined insects crawling under his skin and he harmed himself badly by trying to kill them. He was in hospital for six months because his mother could not cope with his behaviour and on release he was given accommodation in sheltered housing. She visits him daily to help him with the cooking and cleaning and James started painting again when he went to an art class run by a local charity. Although he still hears voices he has learned with the help of medication to control his thoughts and cope with his illness.

Of all the mental illnesses, schizophrenia is probably the one that gets the most media coverage. While the media tend to associate it with violence, many sufferers are timid and sensitive people. The main misconception is that the sufferer has a split personality, the Greek *schizo* meaning split and *phrenia* meaning mind. Schizophrenia really means being separated from one's mind. Many sufferers experience auditory hallucinations, some can experience visual and tactile hallucinations and delusions. The film *A Beautiful Mind* told the story of the brilliant Nobel Prize winning mathematician John Nash, plagued by hallucinations and delusions.

Martin was a bus driver five years ago. One day, someone jumped in front of his bus and died, after Martin's desperate attempt to stop in time. He was consumed with guilt. Even though he was given counselling, he was not able to sleep and kept having flashbacks. His GP gave him sleeping tablets, but they could not stop him having nightmares. His company gave him time off to recover and after three months he went back to work, but even shadows from the tree and falling leaves would cause him to have a panic attack. After a few days he gave up his job. He became depressed and this caused him to lose confidence. Fortunately, a friend told him about a charity wanting volunteers, so Martin is now doing voluntary work.

I learn interesting and sometimes astonishing things from my work. I did a course on different types of mental illness. One of the case studies involved a teenager who suffers from depression, feeling that everything in her life is beyond her control. She worries about not being able to pass her exams and letting her parents down and thinks the only thing she has control over is her weight. She diets excessively until she becomes anorexic. Sometimes, she feels so depressed that she wants to take her own life. Her parents feel helpless. They cannot make her see a way out of this. This teenager's predicament reminded me greatly of the experience of a university friend.

Her family came to England when she was eleven. She was sad to have to leave her friends behind. She spoke little English when she first arrived and, even though the teachers did their best to help her, she felt very isolated in school. Also, she had to help out in her parent's shop after school and she had little chance of making friends. Her only consolation was food. She put on some weight and that made her self-conscious. One day, when one of her relatives commented that she had put on weight, she was upset and determined to lose weight.

Being the eldest child of four children, she felt a lot of pressure on her shoulders. She felt she had to do well and go to university to set a good example for her younger brothers and sisters. Her parents could not drive so they desperately needed her to pass her driving test to help them to run the business. When she failed her driving test, she was devastated, feeling she had let them down badly. Being young, she was not good at handling failure, became depressed and thought she would kill herself if she failed her A levels. There was much pain, but she could not tell people how she was feeling, so she kept a diary.

It was only after she passed her driving test and her 'A' levels that she regained her confidence and she was able to beat anorexia with the help of a counsellor. We became friends at our first year at university. It was in our final year at university, she was able to show me her diary and share her experience with me. At the time, I did not really appreciate what she went through. Now I have a much better understanding of the illness.

Postnatal depression is mainly caused by hormonal changes

after the birth. Other contributing factors can be difficulties with birth or problems with the baby's feeding or sleeping, not lack of ability to bond with the baby. The physical demands of looking after a baby and the lack of sleep make it more difficult to cope with the negative emotions. Some of the symptoms can be physical, such as nausea and dizziness. With the help of a GP, most women recover within months but some take years to recover. Many women find it difficult to seek help because they think it is admitting to being a bad mother. Some fear their child may be taken away if they are not able to cope. Fortunately, such celebrities as Melinda Messenger and Brooke Shields have talked openly about their experience of postnatal depression, helping to remove the stigma attached to the illness.

Obsessive compulsive disorder is common. Most of us have some degree of obsessiveness and compulsiveness in our character. David Beckham has spoken about his obsession with making things line up properly. Obsessions are involuntary thoughts such as fear of dirt, germs or contamination, fears of acting out violent or aggressive thoughts. The main features are: They are automatic, frequent, upsetting and difficult to control. Compulsions are actions people take to reduce the anxiety that comes from an obsession, common ones being excessive cleaning and washing, checking, arranging and ordering. An interesting description for people with OCD is an 'imperfect perfectionist'. Howard Hughes, the millionaire American director and aviator, became so obsessed with being contaminated by germs in later life that he became a virtual prisoner in his own home.

The mentally ill have a much more difficult time and take longer to recover than people with physical illness. Firstly, they are less likely or willing to seek help, often because they have no insight into their illness. Some find it too embarrassing to see their GP or think that their GP can only help with physical health problems. Secondly, diagnosis is very difficult. There is no simple test such as a blood test or urine test that can be used to detect the illness. Brain scans can be used to detect brain damage, but not chemical imbalance. Diagnosis is usually carried out by a psychiatrist by observation of behaviour. Sometimes a patient can exhibit different symptoms at different times and many may be given several diagnoses. The physical symptoms of depression, such as lethargy, can be misdiagnosed as a physical illness. Doctors are reluctant to give a diagnosis to children and young persons, especially for schizophrenia because such a stigmatising label may have a serious impact on the person's education and future career.

Thirdly, the medication can have undesirable side effects and psychological therapies can be difficult to access, although great advancements were made in the early 1950s when the neuroleptic drugs were developed (these act on the nervous system to reduce the psychotic symptoms). Some drugs have some unpleasant side-effects such as increased appetite, tiredness, dry mouth, shakiness, dizziness and stomach upsets. Patients on the drug Clozapine need to take regular blood tests because it may cause a dangerous decrease of white blood cells. Some medication may induce diabetes.

Patients may have to try different medications to find one that suits them.

Psychological therapies are also used to treat mental illness. The most common ones are counselling, psychotherapy and Cognitive Behaviour Therapy (CBT). Access to psychological therapies is not easy. Due to a shortage of trained psychologists, there is often a waiting list of over one year. The NHS has developed two internet CBT courses: Beat the Blue and Fear Fighter to make it more widely available. The licence of the software has to be purchased by the council accessing them depends on a postcode lottery.

Lastly, the lack of support from family, friends, community, workplace and society can be a big barrier to recovery. Support is not easy. Carers provide emotional support, some take responsibility with finance and making sure the patient takes medication and keeps medical and other appointments. People suffering from depression generally feel lethargic, lack motivation and confidence, so carers need to be understanding, calm and positive. Psychotics can exhibit aggression, paranoid ideas and strange behaviour, so living with them is exhausting. Severe mental illness has led to many families break-ups, ostracisation by the community and sackings.

Recovery can mean different things to different people. Some people feel to be 'cured' of mental illness means freedom from medication but this can lead to relapses. Most people accept that recovery often means freedom from symptoms with the help of medication and therapies. Recovery does not necessarily mean going back to the life they led before the illness. Very often, people have to change and learn to follow a different way of life.

Rates of recovery vary individually. For most people, the road to recovery tends to be erratic with fallbacks and restarts. Not being accepted by society is a big barrier to recovery. Many people lose confidence, self-esteem and ability to concentrate as a result of the illness. They have to re-learn these skills as part of their recovery. There is one piece of good news: Research shows that early intervention can play a part in the level of recovery made. Early treatment tends to produce a faster recovery rate.

Self management, a support system where an individual manages his own illness and treatment, is a particularly useful tool for recovery. Individuals need to have insight into their illness, need to know what happens when they are ill, need to recognise early warning signs of relapse and need to plan what to do if they should have a relapse. Self management works particularly well with bipolar patients. Research has shown that people who have received self management training have significantly increased the time between manic episodes.

From my own experience and through working with carers, I found the problems with getting services from the mental health system, and trying to work with professionals, can be as difficult to cope with as dealing with the sufferers' symptoms and behaviour.

The mental health system can seem like a maze because there are different services provided by different areas of the NHS. The biggest problem for someone new to the service is finding out where or who to get help from. Finding the entrance to the maze can seem like an impossible task. Even when you manage to get inside the system, the services can be disjointed and inconsistent. One of the most problematic areas is when someone is discharged from the hospital. Sometimes families are not consulted or informed when someone is discharged and sometimes the care manager in the community health team is not given the relevant information.

Carers often find it difficult getting information about the person they care for. Confidentiality is the biggest barrier between health services, staff and family. For health professionals, confidentiality is a basic aspect of their relationships with their patients. They need to keep in mind that patients have a right to decide what information about themselves should be shared with their family. Without the patients' consent, professionals cannot give information to carers. However, there is nothing to stop families providing information to professionals. It is often useful for professionals to know what the person was like before they developed mental illness. When they are recovering, patients may be more willing for the professionals to share information with their families.

Since Jeff's admission into the mental health system in 2007, I have noticed a gradual improvement in the help and support given to families in my local NHS Trust. There is more information to help carers to understand how the systems work, and carers are now encouraged to attend ward rounds and get involved with care planning. The NHS trust is also emphasising the need for staff to work with families as partners in care.

Mentally ill people are among the various examples of severely disabled people of exceptional talent whose stories are told in chapter 14. There we see how they can be a great inspiration to both carers and cared for.

Part 3

Challenges and Achievements

Chapter 13

Unsung Heroes

Life, misfortunes, isolation, abandonment,
poverty, are battlefields which have their heroes;
obscure heroes sometimes greater than the
illustrious heroes.
Victor Hugo, *Les Miserables*

I have met many carers who devoted their lives to caring for others. Their experiences have moved me and inspired me. Here, I am going to write about some carers who have sacrificed their careers, relationships, freedom and health to care for the people they love.

Many carers do not recognise themselves as carers. It took me a long time to realise that I was a carer because I thought the word signified a profession. I see myself as a mother to Emma and a wife to Jeff, rather than a carer to them. To clarify the group of people I am going to describe in this chapter, I shall use the definition used in the Government's Carers Strategy 'Carers at the heart of 21st century families and communities' published in June, 2008: 'A carer spends a significant proportion of their life providing unpaid support to family or potentially friends. This could be caring for a relative, partner or friend who is ill, frail, disabled or has mental health or substance misuse problems.' Most people in this category do not see themselves as carers because their main role in the relationship means more to them; their role as parent, partner, sibling, relative or friend.

There are six million carers in the UK according to a survey done by the charity Carers UK in June 2007. Together their work is worth £87 billion. The responsibility of caring can fall on anyone – young, old, male, female, rich or poor. About two-thirds of carers are female. 70 percent of those cared for are 65 or over. Most carers live with the person they care for. Although no two carers' experiences are the same, the physical and psychological effects on them of caring are similar.

Research carried out for Carers Week in June 2007 has revealed the far-reaching effects of looking after a loved one across all aspects of a carer's life. The survey asked 3,500 carers about a range of issues, including relationships, health, career and finances. The findings highlight the knock-on effects which caring can have on different areas of life. Contending with emotional or financial difficulties can lead to health problems, such as high levels of stress or depression. In addition, many carers are isolated and do not know where to turn for support.

One of the most difficult challenges carers have to cope with is the impact on their relationships, with two-thirds of those surveyed saying their relationships had suffered as a result of their caring responsibilities. The effects are both emotional and physical, with six in ten reporting they had little quality time with their partners and a similar number saying that their sex lives had taken a back seat directly as a result of their caring role. When carers did get time to relax, more than a fifth used it to catch up on their sleep.

Caring can also lead to financial difficulties, with more than two-thirds saying they were financially worse off as a result of caring. Financial problems can follow when carers' careers are neglected, according to 57 per cent of those questioned. These problems were mainly caused by reduced promotion and training prospects. Almost two-thirds of those surveyed said they felt a loss of identity as a direct result of their caring role. Three quarters had not had a regular break from caring in the past 12 months and 38 per cent had not had a single day off.

Young carers are more likely to be bullied at school because of the stigma attached to disability and because of their lack of progress at school. When asked to describe their experience of being a carer, most chose 'stressful' (74 per cent), and 'demanding' (71 per cent). Despite the challenges of the role, nearly one third of the carers also felt it was 'rewarding'.

My understanding of the burden of caring for someone occurred at the age of five when my grandmother suffered a severe stroke. At the time, she was living with my parents, me and my two sisters, and my mother was pregnant at the time. My grandmother was an independent and fastidious lady. I have fond memories of her taking me to the park, to the market and to the cinema. After the stroke, she lost her mobility and speech and she found it difficult to cope. My mother had to look after my grandmother as well as three young children. Sometimes when my grandmother wanted help and it was delayed, she would scream and throw things at the wall. It was very distressing for all of us. It must have been difficult for my mother. My grandmother died not long after my brother's birth. The only comfort that my mother had was knowing that the birth of my brother, the first boy in the family, brought much joy to my grandmother.

Caring for someone with severe disability can lead to the split up of the family unit. Jan Greenman's story about her son Luke in her book *Life at the Edge* tells of the family being torn apart by Luke's behaviour brought on by Attention Deficit Hyperactive Disorder (ADHD) and Asperger's Syndrome. Luke was born on the same day as Emma (6th December 1991). Jan has had a much harder time than I have; she described Luke as hell on two legs. Luke smashes up the furniture, has physically hurt Jan and his sister, and has run away from home. This extreme behaviour makes it impossible for Jan to have a social life. Luke's father walked out, leaving Jan to cope on her own and she had to give up her career as a successful businesswoman.

Families can lose contact. Michelle and her husband had a happy retirement life together. Michelle, at first, got on well with her husband's daughter and her family. She adores her step grandchildren. But five years ago her husband had a mental breakdown and was diagnosed as being bipolar. Michelle had to cope with this without support from the daughter, who would not allow contact with the grandchildren.

Statistical surveys show that a high percentage of people living in areas of poverty have an illness or disability, and they are especially disadvantaged. I met Sarah and Janette at a training course and their family finance was greatly affected by their caring roles. It is obvious that illness and disability greatly reduce the person's ability to work, but it also reduces their family members' ability to work. Both Sarah's husband and her son are mentally ill. Sarah is divorced from her husband because she could not cope with his violent behaviour. Her son suffers from schizophrenia and his behaviour can be unpredictable. Sarah used to work in a school but had to give up work when her son had a bad spell. She also has a young daughter to look after. She receives Carers Allowance but it is not sufficient. She has a part time job cleaning but, because of the 16 hour limit for claiming Carers Allowance, her earnings are limited.

Janette had an idyllic life, living in a five-bedroomed house in a desirable part of town. Her husband had a thriving business and had a happy life with lots of friends. But after her children were born, things began to change. Janette has two sets of twins, all boys, all of them with learning difficulties and behavioural problems. As the boys became teenagers, Janette's husband could not cope with the demands of the children and left. Janette had to move to a smaller house with the children. She does not receive any help from her husband, has to rely on the state for help and has little time to herself. But she enjoys singing and occasionally sings in a club. This gives her a chance to meet people and also earn some money.

Caring for someone can be more difficult if the cared for person is far away or the carer does not know how to access services. A friend Lalita has a family living in Sri Lanka. Her mother was an independent woman and enjoyed living on her own, with some help from Lalita's sister occasionally. When the mother became ill in 2007, Lalita's sister became her main carer and Lalita felt guilty for not being able to help out. After a few months, it became too much for Lalita's sister, so she went to Sri Lanka to look after her mother for three months, giving her sister a break. The stress of looking after her mother was compounded by the political instability of the country. There was bombing in Columbo and in nearby towns. When Lalita was in Sri Lanka, one of the buses on the route that she took to the nearest town was blown up. Lalita came home after three months because she had to tend to her own family in England. She made a second trip back in June, but sadly her mother passed away before she could see her.

Two of my friends are special needs teachers working with children who have sight and hearing problems in London. They have come across many parents of such children from ethnic groups with little English who lack understanding of these problems and have difficulty accessing such services as support groups and counselling services. Some children are not diagnosed and some of the parents refuse to have respite services because they believe it is their duty to look after their children all the time.

Over 50 per cent of carers are women because it is traditional for women to take care of the family as mother and wife, but men can do the job just as well. My husband Jeff is a good carer: He is dedicated and patient with Emma. Through the Rett support group meetings and annual conference, I also get to know many other caring and dedicated fathers and brothers. The husband of a friend suffering from severe post-natal depression helped to look after the baby and another child to give her time to rest. He also encouraged her to see a counsellor. Fortunately, after a few months she recovered and she was able to look after the baby.

Dementia can happen to anyone, even someone with great intellect such as the writer Iris Murdoch. Her husband John Bayley wrote a moving book, *Elegy for Iris*, about his experience of caring for her when diagnosed as suffering from Alzheimer's. The onset of this disease is frightening, similar to the regression period of Rett Syndrome. I remember the fear in Emma's eyes when she started to lose her hand skills and balance, and her anger and frustrations. It is extremely hard for the family of an Alzheimer's sufferer to accept the new person they become.

Sometimes the caring role has to be passed on to another

person. This happened to Steve when his mother died and he became the carer of his brother. Steve's brother was overweight when he was young. He was bullied at school and this affected his confidence. He was also a sickly child, often missing out on school lessons. When he left school, he managed to get a job. One evening he was robbed and attacked. He was badly hurt and he had a spell in hospital. When he came out he became agorophobic and he had to stay with his mother. He then went into a downward spiral, gave up his job and became an alcoholic. When Steve's mother died, his brother could not look after himself and Steve has to help him with shopping and sometimes cooking.

Looking after someone with mental illness can be exhausting. As well as providing emotional support, encouragement and reassurance, some carers become responsible for finance and for making sure the cared for take medication and keep medical and other appointments. Some carers have to put up with verbal and physical abuse. The unpredictability of the person's behaviour is soul-destroying and lack of respite facilities is one of the major problems for carers. Some carers cannot take holidays or take time off to visit family or friends. The stigma attached to mental illness can isolate carers from the community and from society as a whole.

The age of the carer can affect the person's ability to care. The very young and the very old find it much more difficult to cope. As already noted, a child carer's educational progress can suffer. Sally, 14 years old, looks after her mother who suffers from Multiple Sclerosis, and her 11-year-old sister. She gets up early to prepare breakfast for her mother and at lunch time, she either goes home to check that her mother is OK or phones her. In the evening she cooks and does the housework as well as her homework. Sally has little time to herself, and seldom goes out with her friends. She has to take on the caring role because there is no one else to do it. She started caring at 13 when her mother's illness meant she could not cope with normal household chores. Sally takes on the caring role because she loves her mother and sister, and says that will not leave home and be independent, and she that will have further education locally.

Many older carers have their own health problems. They worry about not being able to continue caring when they become ill. If they are looking after a younger person such as their child, they have to think about making provisions for the person when they are no longer able to care. Recently, an 86-year-old man suffocated his wife because he could not bear to see her suffering so much pain. The benefit system is different for people of a pensionable age. The local carer centre or Citizens Advice Bureau can advise on benefits.

However, there are some older carers managing remarkably well. In May 2010 aged 81, Anne Ravenscroft won the Daily Mail Carer of the Year award for devoting 46 years looking after her daughter Heidi who suffers from Rett Syndrome. Heidi's early development and regression were similar to that of Emma and other Rett girls. In the earlier years there was little knowledge about Rett Syndrome. Heidi did not get diagnosed until her 20s. Anne was Heidi's main carer until she developed cancer in her late 60s. Happily, she made a full recovery and was able to continue caring. In 2005, her husband had a heart attack and Anne had to nurse him back to health as well as caring for Heidi. The amazing thing about Anne is her attitude. She does not think of Heidi as a burden, or consider caring as a chore. Heidi needs her and that is why she takes care of her.

Some carers have to put up with the ignorant comments and aggressive behaviour of others because they are living with someone who is disabled. It is astounding to see these types of unacceptable conduct not only from ignorant juveniles but also from some so-called edgy comedians. How sad it is to see someone has to steep so low to mock people with Down's Syndrome in order to get a few laughs.

The tragic story of Fiona Pilkington highlighted the seriousness of these types of crimes. Fiona suffered years of abuse from her neighbours because of her daughter Francesca's learning disability. Her local council and the police failed to protect her and her family from the daily abuse. Her despair drove her to kill herself and her daughter in a car. I do hope there will be new legislation in the future to stop this type of hate crime from occurring.

Difficulty in accessing services is a common source of distress to carers. Sometimes this can motivate them to start up their own charity. Yvonne Milne is the founder of the Rett Syndrome Association UK. Yvonne's daughter Claire was diagnosed with RS in 1984, a condition almost unheard of at the time. Yvonne was a college lecturer before she gave up work to start the association, starting with a kitchen table, and with no financial help from the council or government. She did receive, however, help from Ann Worthington of the In Touch Trust and received a donation from a local charity. She worked single-handedly for the first six months, being the chairman, secretary and treasurer. Over a number of months, Ann Worthington put her in touch with a few families with children who had been tentatively diagnosed.

In October 1985, The RSAUK held their first get-together and Dr Andreas Rett came to the inaugural meeting at his own expense. At a chance meeting with Harry Secombe, Yvonne asked him to be the patron and he accepted. As the association grew, Yvonne managed to find people to take over the roles of secretary and treasurer. She also managed to get a number of prominent members of the medical profession to become advisors. Yvonne was awarded the MBE in 1997 for her work and today RSAUK has over 1000 members and a staff of six people. Its patrons include Gloria Hunniford, Ann Clwyd MP, Jon Snow and Evelyn Glennie – more about Evelyn in chapter 14.

Experience of poor services from the health system and of the ignorant attitudes of professionals can be upsetting for the families of disabled children. I recall a conversation with Dr Brian Stratford about how he became involved with the Down's Syndrome Association when I met him in China. His interest originated when his daughter Philippa was born with Down's Syndrome in 1965. This is Brian's recollection of the moment when a nurse gave him the news: That stupid bloody nurse came and she said, "She's Mongolian." I shouted at her. I said, "That word is an ethnic description, not a medical condition." I said, "What my daughter has is Down's Syndrome." Philippa died at the age of nine in an accident. Her life changed Brian's attitude towards disability. In his own words, he stopped being a cold, hard-nosed scientist and concerned himself with human values.

Despite the difficulties faced by many carers, caring can be a rewarding experience. It can bring the carer and the cared for person's relationship closer. It can strengthen the carer's character. It can improve the carer's skills and knowledge. To overcome the difficulties of caring, carers need to have a coping strategy. The survival guide in chapter 15 explains how to develop a coping strategy.

If they are to survive these obstacles, if they are to take arms against a sea of troubles and some of the life-enhancing rewards we have seen in this chapter, we will need the survival guide in chapter 15. But meanwhile, it will be salutary to look at some of the extraordinary achievers among the severely physically and mentally handicapped.

Chapter 14

Inspirations

*Now there are diversities of gifts,
but the same Spirit.*
1 Corinthian chapter 12, verse 4

When we feel dissatisfied with our lives, or have to cope with misfortunes, we can get solace and inspiration by considering the achievements of the severely disabled. They remind us that some of the most extraordinary gifts have been born of adversity.

Sport
If we were asked to name a sports person, someone with disability would not immediately come to mind. We tend to associate sports with fitness, strength, speed and agility and we tend to neglect the less obvious but equally important qualities such as commitment and persistence.

The wheelchair is the symbol for disability. People think that wheelchair users cannot do much. However, the Paralympics show us that wheelchair users can perform amazing feats. Tanni Grey-Thompson is considered to be one of the most successful Paralympic athletes in the UK. She was born in

Cardiff in 1969. She has spina bifida. During her competing career, she has won 16 Paralympic medals including 11 gold medals. She was awarded the MBE in 2000, and the DBE in 2005.

One of my colleagues was a wheelchair user. Talking to him one lunchtime, I discovered that he was a member of the Jubilee Sailing Trust and that he went sailing regularly on the Lord Nelson. Out of curiosity, I looked up sailing for the disabled and I came across Vinny Lauwers who is the first disabled person to sail solo, non-stop and unassisted around the world.

Vinny Lauwers lost his ability to walk after a motorcycle accident when he was 22. He made a remarkable recovery, but lost his love for life for a while. One thing that kept him going was his dream to sail around the world one day. As a 14-year-old boy he sailed with a crew from Melbourne to Sydney. In May 2001 he was awarded the International Disabled Sports Person of the Year award at the World Sports Awards in Monaco.

About one third of the way through the gruelling course of the Oxfam TrailWalker challenge in 2003, I was overtaken by a man with a prosethic leg and arm. Later, I discovered this man was Chris Moon. He had been an army officer specialising in clearing landmines. In Mozambique he was blown up walking in a supposedly cleared area, losing his lower right arm and right leg. He survived through sheer determination and fitness.

Less than a year after leaving hospital he completed the London Marathon. He has done numerous marathons and some of the world's toughest ultra-marathons including the Great Sahara Run and the 135-mile run through Death Valley in the USA. He has written a book called *A Step Beyond* and he is now working as a motivational speaker.

Music

I mentioned in chapter 6 that I have been inspired by Emma's love of music to learn to play the piano. One of the pieces that I enjoy playing, but find hard to master is *Fur Elise* by Beethoven. Curious about who Elise was, I went on the internet to search for her. Who was she? I knew it was a famous piece of piano music but I was stunned to find how popular it is with young people: Numerous people posting themselves playing it on YouTube, for a dedicated website for people to tell their story about learning to play the piece, written almost 200 years ago by a deaf composer.

Beethoven was born in Bonn in 1770. In his youth, he made a living as a pianist, violinist and music teacher. He was a composer from an early age. His hearing deteriorated in his early twenties. He used a special rod attached to the soundboard on a piano that he could bite – the vibrations would then transfer from the piano to his jaw to increase his perception of the sound. Despite his disability, Beethoven went on to compose some of the best loved music we hear today. His musical genius was not diminished by deafness or depression.

Another musician who had to overcome deafness is Evelyn Glennie. Evelyn was born in Aberdeen, started to lose her hearing at the age of eight, and by the age of 12 was profoundly deaf. After that, she took up percussion instruments. In 1982, at the Royal Academy of Music she was awarded the prestigious Shell/LSO Gold Medal for Percussion and Piano. She became a solo percussionist and she now tours the world to give performances. She also works as a motivational speaker and composes music for TV productions.

She owns over 1800 musical instruments from all over the world, and she regularly plays barefoot for both live performances and recordings to get a better feel for the music. She was awarded the OBE in 1993 and the DBE in 2007. She is a patron of the Rett Syndrome Association UK and I had the honour of seeing her perform and meeting her in a RSAUK fundraising event in March 2009.

I find learning to play the piano a difficult task, requiring the co-ordination of the eyes, ears and hands. It is astonishing that some people who do not have sight can create such wonderful music as Ray Charles. He was born in Albany, Georgia, USA. He started to lose his sight around five and became totally blind by seven. He attended the Florida School for Deaf and Blind where he learned to play the piano and started on a musical career as a pianist for different bands. In 1947, he started recording music, his second album being a big success in 1949. His fame grew and he performed all over the world, but he had a troubled life – addicted to heroin and arrested three times. His other passion apart from music was civil rights for black people, and he was a supporter of Martin Luther King. Ray Charles was a prolific musician, producing many albums, and he won 17 Grammy Awards. His music is still being enjoyed by millions and the film *Ray* of 2005 tells his story and celebrates his achievements. Sadly, he died before the film was opened.

Art

Before Emma's diagnosis, we had thought that she might have autism or some sort of brain injury, so I had done a lot of reading on the subjects. When I saw a television programme about a young boy called Stephen Wiltshire, I was fascinated by his amazing drawing talent. Stephen is autistic but he has an extraordinary memory of details which enables him to draw complicated buildings from memory. He only has to look at a building such as Charing Cross station or the skyscrapers in New York and he can draw these buildings with all the fine details. I read about Stephen's story in various newspapers and magazines. The last time I heard he was attending an art college. His communication skills had improved and he was enjoying life as an art student.

The first time I saw a painting of Richard Wawro on the internet, I was bowled over by its rich colours. Richard was born in 1952 and was three years old when his parents were told that he was moderately to severely retarded, showing autistic behaviour. He required surgery for cataracts on both eyes during childhood. Aged six he entered a Children's Centre where he was introduced to drawing with crayons and his immense talent was immediately apparent.

Richard used wax crayons to paint his pictures, producing them from memory, a talent similar to Stephen Wiltshire's. His works have been described as an "incredible phenomenon rendered with the precision of a mechanic and the vision of a poet". Now he is known worldwide and has sold over 1000 pictures in over 100 exhibitions. One of his exhibitions was opened by Margaret Thatcher when she was Minister of Education, she owns several of his pictures as did the late Pope John Paul II.

One of the best known artists for using rich colours was Vincent Van Gogh, who suffered from depression. He was born in Groot-Zundert, Holland, in 1853, son of a pastor. He studied in Belgium. His early paintings were sombre-toned, but later his work was influenced by the Impressionists when he went to live and work in France. In 1886 he went to Paris to join his brother Theo and he met Pissarro, Monet and Gauguin. He went to Arles in the south of France to set up a school of art and was joined by Gauguin later. His nervous temperament made him a difficult companion and night-long discussions combined with painting all day undermined his health. After cutting part of an ear off, Van Gogh's mental health deteriorated and he was sent to the asylum in Saint-Remy for treatment.

During the last three years of his life, he produced his finest works while struggling against madness and ill health. His brushstroke technique became more impassioned, his colours more intense and the contents more dramatic. In May 1890, he went to live in Auvers-sur-Oise under the supervision of

Dr. Gachet. Two months later he was dead at the age of 37, having shot himself "for the good of all".

Literature
The three authors mentioned in this section all used personal experience of disability and mental illness as subjects in their work.

Helen Adams Keller was born with full sight and hearing on 27 June 1880 in Alabama, USA. When Helen was 19 months old, she fell ill with a fever which left her both blind and deaf. She became a very difficult child, smashing dishes and lamps and terrorising the whole household with her screaming and temper tantrums. Anne Sullivan became Helen's teacher in 1887. She used finger movements to teach Helen to spell words on her hands. Under Anne's patient and inspired guidance, Helen learned to read and write but her speech was limited to sounds that only Anne and others close to her could understand.

Helen moved on to the Cambridge School for Young Ladies in 1896 and in the Autumn of 1900 entered Radcliffe College, becoming the first deafblind person to have ever enrolled at an institution of higher learning. Helen's first book, *The Story of My Life*, published in 1903, has since become a classic. On 28 June 1904 Helen graduated with a BA. She wrote *Out of the Dark* in 1913. Later, Helen travelled the world with Anne to do lecture tours, speaking of her experiences and beliefs to enthralled crowds. She died in 1968. With the help of Anne Sullivan, through her writings, lectures and the way she lived her life, Helen Keller had shown millions of people how to triumph over severe disability.

Tennessee Williams's work was focused heavily on his experiences of mental illness, alcoholism and drug addiction. He was born in 1911 in Columbus, Mississippi, USA. His early family life was full of tension. His sister Rose suffered from schizophrenia and his mother had her lobotomised. She was the inspiration for the plays *The Glass Menagerie* and *Suddenly Last Summer*. Williams himself suffered from depression, and was addicted to prescription drugs and alcohol, and feared that he would become mentally unstable like his sister. Several plays were made into films. He won two Pulitzer Prizes and four New York Drama Critics' Circle Awards.

Christy Brown, the Irish poet, was born with cerebral palsy in 1932. He was the tenth child of a Dublin bricklayer. He was unable to control his speech and body, apart from his left foot. For some years he was met with ignorance and embarrassment. Fortunately, his mother was a steadfast champion. One day, he used his left foot to pick up his sister's chalk and scribbled on the floor. His family was excited by this achievement. His mother wrote the letter A on the floor and Christy managed to copy it after a few trials: that was the start of his ability to communicate. At the age of five, using his left foot, Christy wrote the autobiographical novel *Down All The Days*. He has also written other novels and published poetry.

Science

The theoretical physicist Professor Stephen Hawking is probably the world's most iconic wheelchair user. He was born in Oxford in 1942, and while studying at Cambridge University he was laid low by motor neuron disease, gradually losing his ability to walk and speak. By 1974 he was unable to feed himself or get out of bed. With the help of a voice synthesizer he was able to communicate and in 1988, he published his magnum opus, *A Brief History of Time,* which became a bestseller.

The 1994 winner of the Nobel Memorial Prize in Economic Sciences, John Nash was the subject of the film *A Beautiful Mind*. It told the story of this brilliant mathematician and economist, and his struggle with paranoid schizophrenia. It showed how hallucinations and delusions can dominate someone's thinking and make them lose touch with reality. For the purpose of the film, John Nash was shown suffering from visual hallucinations, but in real life he suffered from auditory hallucinations. Born in 1928, he has worked on game theory, differential geometry, partial differential equations and economic theories. In 1994, he shared the Nobel Memorial Prize in Economic Sciences with two other game theorists. His theories are still used today in market economics, accounting and military theory.

Kim Peek who died in 2009 was the inspiration for the film *Rainman*. Although Kim had the same incredible mathematic skills and photographic memory as Raymond in that film, he did not have Raymond's autism. He was born with macrocephaly, and damage to the brain; the part that connects the two hemispheres of the brain was missing. According to Kim's father, Fran, at the age of 16 months had developed an extraordinary memory. He read books, memorised them, and then placed them upside down on the shelf to show that he had finished reading them, a practice he still maintains. He read a book in about an hour and remembers 98.7% (according to the internet) of everything he has read. He could memorise vast amounts of information in subjects ranging from history, literature, geography, and numbers to sports, music, and dates. The 'Walking Google' could recall the content of some 12,000 books from memory.

Politics

Franklin Delano Roosevelt was born in 1882 in Hyde Park, New York, to a wealthy family. He became the 32nd president of the USA in 1933, and he was a central figure of the 20th century during the period of depression and World War Two, elected to four terms. He went to Harvard University and was trained as a lawyer. In 1921, he contracted an illness believed to be Polio at the time, which caused him permanent paralysis from the waist down. His disability did not prevent him from being president and doing an extremely important and demanding job.

David Blunkett was born in Sheffield on 6th June 1947 and lived in Hillsborough. He was blind at birth and he had to leave the family home to board at the Sheffield School for the Blind on Manchester Road at the age of four. In 1963, just after David's sixteenth birthday, he joined the Labour Party.

He went to Sheffield University to study Politics and his first job was with the East Midlands Gas Board where he taught industrial relations and politics and was also a member of Unison. He entered the House of Commons as the Member of Parliament (MP) for Sheffield Brightside in 1987. He was the Shadow Secretary of State for Education and Employment until the General Election of 1997. He held the position of Shadow Secretary of State for Education between 1994 and 1995. He relies heavily on his guide dog which accompanies him everywhere.

Jack Ashley was the UK's first totally deaf MP. One of three children born to a poor family in Widnes, Jack Ashley was only five when his father died. He left school at 14 to work in a factory, became a shop steward at 20 and a local councillor at 23. He won a scholarship to study at Oxford and then Cambridge. In 1966 he became the MP for Stoke-on-Trent. He became totally deaf at 45 after a routine ear operation went wrong.

Jack Ashley established himself as an MP who was combative and outspoken in his fight against a wide range of social injustices. As he became increasingly famous as a passionate advocate for disabled rights, he became President of the Royal National Institute for the Deaf. In 1993 his hearing was partially restored by a cochlea implant, an electronic device which stimulates the nerves in the inner ear. Today he is a member of the house of Lords, still campaigning for disabled rights.

What these inspirational stories leave with us is the wonderful compensation nature can provide for the severely disabled: Sometimes extraordinary gifts unattainable by the 'normal'.

Chapter 15

A Survival Guide

Life is a journey that must be travelled, no matter
how bad the road condition and accommodation.
Oliver Goldsmith (1730–74)

A journey is often used as an analogy for life. It has a beginning
and an end; a traveller can take different paths, use different
modes of transport, choose different accommodations,
experience different climates and weather changes and meet
different people along the way. For some carers, life is often an
uphill struggle, having to cope with unfamiliar situations and
dealing with unexpected setbacks. As we saw in chapter 13,
carers have varied caring experiences, but their needs are
similar. Different people have different ways of coping and
some cope better than others. How can you learn to cope?

On 26th July 2003, I took part in the Oxfam TrailWalker
challenge with three colleagues – Martin, Nik and Carl. The
challenge was to complete a 100 km walk along the South
Downs in less than 30 hours. The route is used by the Ghurka
soldiers for military training. It was a wet and rainy day, but
we managed to complete the walk in 23 hours and 49

minutes. I came away with some cuts and bruises from a fall, a few blisters, two black toenails and two extremely swollen feet – very tired but exalted.

What helped us were: Good preparation, good maps, physical fitness, a positive mental attitude and support. Oxfam provided excellent maps giving directions, gradients of landscape, timing and location of checkpoints. We had been doing fitness training for a few months in preparation for the walk and we were in good shape: Well equipped with clothing for bad weather, blister plasters, painkillers, head lights, torches, spare batteries, and spare boots. Jeff and a colleague Alan provided the much needed support, meeting us at checkpoints to give us food and drinks, chairs to sit on, sympathy and encouragement. Overcoming the fear of unfriendly looking bulls in fields, the worry about having another fall, the pains in my feet and legs, refusing to give up was what that mental attitude was all about.

Getting Informed

Carers need a map as much as walkers do. Where do you start? Which is the best route? What is the destination? The first thing carers need to know is the condition of the people they care for. This information is not readily available and you need to work hard to obtain it. With both Emma and Jeff, the lack of understanding of their conditions was the most distressing part. It took nearly two years to get a diagnosis for Emma. With Jeff, it took a long time for his depression to emerge and for me to understand his condition. Things become easier when you know from what the person is suffering. The news may be devastating, but it helps you on your way.

The GP is the first port of call whether the person is having physical or mental problems. He will guide you. The internet is a good source of information. The local council website is particularly useful for services available near where you live. Local libraries and community centres are also good sources of information.

Local carers' centres are a good place to start: They can provide emotional support, advice on benefits and practical help; some can help with respite and sitting services. The Citizens Advice Bureau will help with legal matters. Charities can provide emotional and practical support.

The local council is responsible for social care, education and nurseries, and will advise on benefits available. Central government provides benefits such as Carers Allowance and Disability Living Allowance.

Appendix C contains the names and addresses of many organisations that can provide support to carers.

Health and Fitness
Good health is particularly important for carers because of the physical and mental demands. Regular exercise can reduce stress levels, improve mood and reduce the chances of depression and boost the immune system. About 30 minutes a day every day is more effective than working out once or twice

a week. One of the things carers desperately lack is time, so try to walk instead of taking the car or public transport. If it is hard to leave the cared for person at home, try doing exercises such as Tai Chi or Yoga at home or use exercise machines.

Healthy Eating

A good balanced diet is about having the right combination of nourishing food and avoid or cut down on things that are bad for you. We all need a balance of carbohydrates, protein, fat, fibre, vitamins, and minerals to sustain a healthy body. We should avoid highly processed food that have been stripped of bran, fibre, nutrients or have preservatives, high contents of sugar or salt.

Food can give us energy as well as improve our mental and emotional wellbeing. Vitamins and nutrients and dopamine can help people to cope with stress, Taurine can help with calming and Melatonin can aid sleeping. You can find Dopamine in fish, bacon, ham, pulses, potatoes and tomatoes, Taurine in meat, fish, eggs, pulses and nuts, and Melatonin in rice, tomatoes and bananas. Carers need to be disciplined and avoid comfort eating, smoking, alcohol and street drugs. It is best to avoid sleeping tablets.

Getting Support

Your GP will suggest appropriate support. It may come from counsellors, social workers, health workers, charities, family, friends and neighbours.

You may find counselling useful. You can ask your GP to refer you to a counsellor. Family counselling services are also available from the NHS and from organisations such as Relate. An experienced counsellor will talk through your difficulties with you and help you to arrive at decisions for yourself.

I found joining a RS support group and meeting other families in a similar situation an enormous help. You can learn a lot from their experiences. You can join an online support group and 'talk' to other carers on the internet. An advantage of using online support groups is that you can talk to people from all over the world.

Planning Ahead

Most planning tends to be centred on the people we care for. Carers of disabled children need to plan for further education and life beyond that. When disabled children become adults, all the services change. Parents need to spend a lot of time finding the appropriate services such as further education college, respite care and leisure activities. Emma is going through the transition process at present, as I have described, and coping is not easy.

A plan is needed to help the cared for person to recover, build confidence and return to normality if that is possible. It is particularly important if the recovery is going to be long: The time involved in caring and the impact on family finance needs to be considered. Sometimes planning involves making difficult choices. For people with terminal illness or dementia, families have to make important decisions that have an impact on the entire family. It is important to consult people involved and make these decisions jointly.

After discharge from an institution it is important to ensure that there is a home care plan. The health authority is responsible for providing patients' aftercare and for ensuring families have sufficient support, financial and social, to look after the patient at home. Carers are entitled to have an assessment. The tasks faced by a carer need to be identified, as well as the patient's needs.

Making a will is something many people are reluctant to do. It is especially difficult when it is for the cared for person. Their wishes should be recorded and carried out if they are capable of expressing them. They may lose that capacity long before death.

Being Positive
Carers often feel frustrated and angry; I know I do. They feel angry with the person they support for being a burden, with themselves for not coping, with the professionals for not listening or being unhelpful, with the health or social system for not providing the appropriate services, with friends and family for not being supportive, with strangers staring or making hurtful comments, with God for allowing the tragedy to happen to them.

Some of the carers' complaints are justifiable and some are not. Being angry can be counter productive. You need to put yourself in other people's shoes, understand why people behave in the way they do and learn to forgive them, work with them and make the most of the services available.

As described in chapter 13, many carers suffer from ill health or depression. There is a saying: If we cannot change the situation we are in, we can change the way we think about it and learn to cope with it. Learning to accept being a carer is a big milestone. Reluctance to accept it will only make life more difficult for you and the person you care for. The challenges of caring for someone can make us feel helpless and hopeless. The frustration and despair can sometimes be exploited, of course, to drive us to improve the services that we feel let down by, to educate people who do not understand our problems, to set up organisations and facilities. This is what Yvonne Milne and the Stratfords did.

Brenda Munitich has been a full time carer for her husband and her son for over 20 years. She has put the wisdom she has gained into a wonderful book called *The little book of positive thoughts for carers*. More details about this book are in the Bibliography.

Making time to recharge
On that trail, I was able to take a rest at some of the checkpoints and have something to eat. Without these stops I would not have had enough energy to complete the walk. When looking after someone long term, you need time to recharge your batteries.

We are fortunate to have respite care for Emma two nights a

month and, occasionally, Emma goes to a Saturday club. These short breaks enable Jeff and I to go out for a meal or go to the cinema. On the occasional free Saturdays, I go shopping or meet up with a friend. The local councils have a duty to provide respite for people with disability. Some carers' centres and charities provide sitting service and respite care.

Some carers do not make use of these facilities because they do not know about them or they feel guilty about leaving the person they care for with someone else, or they worry about the person not being able to manage. The consequence of not taking time out to rest can leave you tired, emotionally drained and isolated from friends and family. This will affect not only yourself but also the quality of care you can provide.

You can also use the free time to learn something new or make new friends. Some carer centres or community centres run courses on painting, creative writing and pottery classes for a low cost. Some provide alternative therapies and outings. Part of my work is to organise courses for carers. I know how much carers get out of these courses.

Hugh Marriott's book *A selfish pig's guide to caring* shows a refreshing approach to the subject. The main theme is carers need to look after themselves otherwise they cannot provide adequate support for the person they care for. It also deals with difficult subjects such as toileting, bathing and sex. Perhaps its most important contribution to the subject is the humour to be got out of it – reflected in the title.

I find the wonderful poems from the American poet Ella Wheeler Wilcox (1855 – 1919) round up this subject matter nicely.

Laugh and the world laughs with you;
Weep, and you weep alone;
For the sad old earth must borrow its mirth;
It has trouble enough of its own.
('Solitude')

So many gods, so many creeds,
So many paths that wind and wind,
While just the art of being kind
Is all the sad world needs.
('The World's Needs')

Chapter 16

Faith in the Future

Where there is discord, may we bring harmony.
Where there is error, may we bring truth. Where
there is doubt, may we bring faith. Where there is
despair, may we bring hope.
St Francis of Assisi

Margaret Thatcher quoted St Francis of Assis on the steps of 10 Downing Street when she was elected prime minister in 1979. A new government is a time for taking stock and for making new beginnings. There is some uncertainty, and a need for a prayer. I believe this prayer will be equally appropriate for people who are entering a new phase of their life and are uncertain of their future.

For many people who are in the fifth decade of their life, there is a certain amount of trepidation. They worry about their health, their children's future, their finances and growing old and becoming less independent. At the time of writing I am just a few months after the half a century milestone and certainly have more to fear than most people. My main concern is Emma's future. I am not sure what provision there is for her when she leaves full time education. I also worry about Jeff. My biggest fear is about becoming old and frail, and not being able to look after Emma, Jeff or myself.

Fear of the future is a common phobia especially among carers. To overcome the fear, we must have faith in the future, in the government to bring about improvements in health and in social, transport and educational services. We need to have faith in medical researches to bring new treatments and technological advancements to bring new equipments for improving mobility and communication and, most of all, we need to have faith in ourselves to overcome problems and to obtain better services for the people we care for and for ourselves.

Although families with disabled children are still experiencing difficulties with lack of support and lack of facilities, things have improved considerably over the last 30 years. Until the 1960s, the choice for disabled adults and for many disabled children was quite restricted: Either stay in an institution or in a family home. Now there are more options and more support for the relatives of the disabled. Before the 1970s there was no law to give disabled people equal opportunity at work. There were very few facilities for the disabled, such as ramps and disabled toilets, use of braille and sign language in public places. There were no special schools for children with severe learning disabilities. Now every disabled child goes to school, whether mainstream or special.

Attitudes to people with disabilities are improving slowly and opportunities are increasing. Terms such as mental handicap and mental retardation have been replaced by more sympathetic descriptions such as learning disability or learning difficulty. More supportive services are now available. The internet provides opportunities for people to communicate and make friends. Most charities now have their own websites. The travel industry and holiday companies are providing special facilities.

Where the disabled are taught in mainstream schools, there is greater understanding of disability among children and their parents. Some schools have disabled and normal children in the same class, or all children sharing non-academic classes such PE or cookery. Emma went to a special unit within a mainstream school. Her unit joined the other children for assembly, PE, music and cookery classes. At her current school, as described in chapter 6, they have half a day integration with a local comprehensive school.

In chapter 14, I wrote about disabled people's talents and how their contributions enrich our lives. I am pleased to learn that in the 2012 Olympics, disabled people will not only have a chance to show their talents in the Paralympics, they will also have opportunities to demonstrate their talents in arts. As part of the Olympics celebration, London will stage a Cultural Olympiad – a series of events to show the UK's arts and culture to the rest of the world. One of the projects of the Cultural Olympiad is called *Unlimited* which is a disability arts project. Disabled artists from across the UK will be commissioned to showcase their work in dance, music, plays and drama. I believe these shows will challenge people's perception of disability and inspire them.

We are still a long way away from the statement Tony Blair, the Prime Minister made in 1997, that Government policy was directed at creating a society 'in which every citizen is valued and has a chance; in which no one is excluded from the opportunity and the chance to develop their potential'. A lot of progress has been made since the disabled were kept in institutions apart from the community, but there is a lot more to be done if the disabled are to develop their potential.

My greatest hope for Emma's future is in new developments in genetic research. A lot of new advances in the diagnosis and treatment of Rett Syndrome have been made in recent years. There is a possibility of using a drug to reverse the symptoms of Rett Syndrome in the future. Full details of research and recent developments are described in appendix A.

Through my work as a Carer Support Worker and now as a NHS Trust Carer Lead, I have been seeing improvements made to the treatment of mentally ill people. In Jeff's hospital, they now have an information pack for families and they are involving families in the care planning, training staff to work with carers and run support groups for carers.

One of the big barriers to the recovery of the mentally ill is lack of social acceptance. The national movement Time to Change was formed in 2007 to remove the stigma attached to mental illness. The organisation, supported by the Mental

Health Media, and by the organisations Mind and Rethink, is funded by the Lottery Fund and Comic Relief. Its main functions are to organise physical activities for the mentally ill, training for medical students, student teachers and social workers, and to provide help with awareness campaigns.

Mental illness costs British business £26 billion a year. The Government and the leading mental health organisation Sainsbury Centre are working together to help the mentally ill to stay at work or return to work using the 'Beyond Blue' model developed in Australia. This programme gives line managers in businesses the skills, knowledge and confidence to offer the right support to people who are experiencing distress at work. I notice there are already advertisements appearing on television promoting this.

One of the areas that is still lacking is carers' rights. Even now, carers are still having problems in getting time off from work to support the person they care for, to attend hospital appointments, for example: Some carers become so desperate that they have to lie to get time off work. In Australia, they have Carers' Day to enable carers to take time off to support their family. We need some sort of recognition here.

As for carers like myself, things have come a long way. From talking to older carers, I realised there was no recognition for the work they did and there was little help available until 1991 when the Prime Minister, John Major, launched the Caring for Carers strategy. There was little known about carers until the 2001 Census.

What carers constantly demand is information. The government initiative 'A New Deal for Carers' provides training for carers. A consortium made up of Carers UK, Crossroads Caring for Carers, Expert Patient's Programme Community Interest Company (EPP CIC), Partners in Policymaking, and the Princess Royal Trust have developed the Caring with Confidence course which covers seven main areas of caring. The face-to-face training has been tried in a few locations in England and is being rolled out to all regions in the UK via local agencies in 2009. The consortium is making the courses available as self study packs and on the internet. This will be a great help to carers. A number of carers I know have attended a Caring with Confidence course and the feedback was positive. I have completed the online course and I found it flexible and easy to do. It is ideal for carers who have limited time and may have difficulty in attending classes regularly. More details about the course is in appendix C.

One of the biggest problems for me as a carer is lack of recognition from the medical and health professionals who look after Emma and Jeff. Most of them do not understand my needs and are unable or unwilling to give me support. Over the years, I noticed a gradual improvement in attitude. I understand that training for new doctors and nurses now includes working with the families of the patients. Some carer organisations run courses for newly qualified social care professionals. As for professionals who have been working for many years, some councils and NHS Trusts have their own training courses. At the NHS Trust where I work, there is a Family Inclusive Practice training course for staff to learn about carers' needs and working with carers. The most important part of the course is a talk from a carer about his caring experience. It is pleasing to know that some councils and NHS trusts are taking the initiatives to train their staff, but there is a need for a national drive.

The Government launched its national carers' strategy, 'Carers at the heart of 21st century families and communities' in June 2008. It promised to commit £255 million to create additional support for carers. It also set out medium and long-term plans aimed at transforming the way that society treats carers especially the health care professionals. There is an initiative sponsored by the Department of Health called Learning for Change, which is developing a national training and learning resource for professionals working with carers. The project is currently researching and gathering materials from organisations that have already developed their own training courses.

There are decisions about services and pilots of annual health checks for carers in a number of Primary Care Trusts. Other recommendations are: Provide more respite breaks for carers; the raising of awareness among employers that carers have the right to request flexible working; help to get carers back to work; help for young carers to ensure their education is not affected by their caring role; and more accurate data about carers to help future planning.

The new initiatives should benefit all carers in different ways.

Some of them tend to be so bureaucratically detailed that carers are discouraged from making use of them. Some of them are not sufficiently publicised; it is not clear for example how to claim for Carers Allowance and there are thousands of people who are entitled to this benefit and are unaware of the fact. Sometimes money for carers' projects is not ring fenced when it is given to local councils or Primary Care Trusts. This can result in the money being spent on other projects.

A lot more work still needs to be done. But at least new carers will not have to go through the struggle that I went through. I am encouraged enough to hope for a much better future for the cared for and the carers, when those initiatives are clear to all and put into practice.

Eighteen years of being a carer is an epic journey that has left me weary and sometimes frustrated, but it has not diminished my faith and hope. I still have faith in my own ability to manage my life and care for Emma and Jeff, faith in the government and in society as a whole to be caring to those in need, and faith in human intelligence and perseverance to solve the mysteries of nature. I still have hope that Emma will be able to talk to me one day – not in my dreams, but for real.

Appendix A

The Story of Rett Syndrome

In 1966, a paediatrician, Dr Andreas Rett, first noticed some of his girl patients wringing their hands, mouthing and walking with a wide gait. He wrote a report on this strange behaviour which was published in a German medical journal. Dr Rett was born in Furth, Bavaria in 1924. He had studied medicine at the University of Innsbruck. After graduation, he moved to Vienna to start his paediatric training. He was a compassionate man and he had a particular interest in children with disabilities.

His report went unnoticed for almost 20 years. In 1983, a team of Swedish doctors led by Professor Bengt Hagberg noticed similar symptoms in young girls. They found Dr Rett's report and published it in English. The condition was designated Rett Syndrome. Following the publication of the report, RS became better known. Other such cases were so designated.

In 1984 in the UK, Yvonne Milne's daughter Claire was diagnosed as having RS. After Claire's diagnosis, Yvonne founded the Rett Syndrome Association UK (RSAUK) which provides support for parents and promotes awareness. The organisation now has over one thousand members, medical professionals, health workers and teaching professionals. Yvonne was awarded the MBE in 1997 for her tireless efforts.

In 1984, in the US, Kathy Hunter's daughter Stacey was diagnosed with RS. Kathy founded the US Rett Syndrome Association (USRSA) and later the International Rett Syndrome Association (IRSA). Kathy did much to promote awareness of RS. She wrote several books about it and she travelled the world.

The cause of RS is genetic. However, to find the faulty gene that causes RS is like looking for a needle in a haystack. After years of research, there was a breakthrough in the USA. Bill and Maureen Woodcock in Union in Washington have three children, Martin, Tiffany and Erica. Martin and Tiffany are normal, healthy children, Erica has physical and learning disabilities. Maureen tried for years to find out what was wrong with Erica. In 1986 Maureen discovered that she had RS.

Tiffany got married in 1995 and nine months later she gave birth to a healthy six and a half pound baby girl called Paige. Maureen was overjoyed at becoming a grandmother. One day Tiffany rang and asked Maureen what Erica was like when she was five months old; Paige was behaving strangely. Maureen knew this was an ominous question. She told Tiffany about Erica and suggested that Tiffany should take Paige to hospital for tests. When Paige was diagnosed with RS, Maureen was distraught. How could this rare condition affect two generations of the same family? Maureen wanted to know whether this had happened to other families. She logged onto the Rett Net and e-mailed other RS families.

No other families contacted had two RS girls. Dr Caroline Channing of Stanford University noticed Maureen's email and asked for Maureen's family to give gene samples. The results brought surprises – Tiffany has the same X chromosome structure as Erica and Paige. That means Tiffany also has RS, although a very mild form. There was something in her DNA that suppressed the expression of RS symptoms about 85 per cent of the time. The gene samples provided by Erica, Tiffany and Paige were a great help to the researchers. It helped them to reduce the genes they needed to look at by one third.

There were still more surprising discoveries to come from the Woodcock family. Tiffany became pregnant again and she had a boy called Ari. When Ari was born, he was a healthy 8lb baby. He was a passive baby, did not cry and would not suck. A few days after Tiffany took Ari home, she phoned Maureen for help. It was clear that Ari could not suck and he was dehydrated. He was taken to hospital. He had more seizures, reflux and an EEG showed that his brain activities were slowing down. Could Ari have RS? It had been thought that male babies with RS would not survive the first few weeks of pregnancy. The gene samples taken from Ari showed that they had the same structure as Erica, Tiffany and Paige. It was confirmed that Ari had RS.

Despite the problems he suffered, Ari fought heroically for

his life. He made some amazing comebacks from the brink of death – they called him the comeback kid. Ari was a tiny miracle and the information from his genes provided more clues about RS than female genes. With his extraordinary spirit and resilience he managed to live for one year and fifteen days.

In September 1999, a researcher, Ignata Van Veyer at Baylor College of Medicine in Houston, Texas, working on mutation detection asked for a gene sample from a RS patient to use as a control. She observed something completely unexpected from the controlled sample and she asked fellow researcher Ruthie Amir to investigate. So Ruthie and her team carried out mutation detection tests with samples from RS patients and they found that there was an extra band appearing on her Rett samples, but not on the others. Ruthie could not believe her eyes when the first results were in, so this time she wanted to be sure. Soon she was certain it was something to show to Dr Huda Zoghbi. When Dr Zoghbi was with Ruthie, she confirmed that the Rett samples did indeed contain mutation. They were excited – they had worked on this for so many years with many disappointments.

The team screened more patients, carried out more experiments and found more mutations. They knew that they were on the right track. On 30/09/1999, the discovery made by Dr Zoghbi's team, in collaboration with Dr Uta Franke from Stanford University, was announced in a press conference in Houston. RS had been traced to mutations observed in a gene called MECP2 (Metho CPG binding protein 2), which is located in the X chromosome. Publication of their findings appeared in the October 1999 edition of the scientific journal *Nature Genetics*.

The information about the Woodcock family and the research leading to the discovery of Rett Syndrome being caused by the mutation of the MECP2 gene was extracted from the documentary *'silent Angels'* hosted by Julia Roberts in 2000. Julia became involved after she met Abigail Brodsky of Brooklyn in New York, who has Rett Syndrome. She also attended a session at the House of Representatives health committee to make a pledge for funding into research into Rett Syndrome.

In 2006, Coleen Rooney (nee McLoughlin) talked about her adopted sister Rosie who suffers from Rett Syndrome in ITV's *Tonight with Trevor McDonald*. Rosie was fostered by Coleen's parents at the age of two and later they adopted her. They knew she was ill but they did not know how serious it would turn out to be. When Rosie arrived she could crawl, and even though she couldn't use her hands much she would handle toys on her play mat and she could eat. But over a period of time she stopped crawling and regressed. She also started having problems swallowing her food. She would cough and choke and bring food back up as she was trying to eat. Rosie's condition was diagnosed when she was three. Today, both Coleen and Wayne Rooney are involved with the Rett Syndrome Association.

There was also another important development in 1999. Monica Coenraads, mother of a two-year-old Rett girl, co-founded the Rett Syndrome Research Foundation and became the Scientific Director. The aim of the Foundation is to stimulate scientific interest and research in Rett Syndrome.

One of the projects funded by the Foundation was led by Professor Adrian Bird of Edinburgh University. In 2007, the team made a significant breakthrough in finding a cure for Rett Syndrome. The team has made symptoms of Rett Syndrome disappear in mice by activating the MECP2 gene.

In sufferers of Rett Syndrome, MECP2 gene is faulty and 'switched off' in most cells. The scientists studied mice born with the gene switched off. Activating the gene stopped symptoms such as breathing and mobility difficulties. It may be years before this can be applied to humans, but teams all over the world are working on a cure for Rett Syndrome and other MECP2 related conditions such as autism, Angelman's Syndrome, schizophrenia and bipolar. The Rett Syndrome Research Foundation is running the Research to Reality campaign to raise money to find a cure. The latest research news and advice can be found on the website: www.rettsyndrome.org

Appendix B

Chronology of Emma

Age	Date	Test/Assessment/Treatment
1 day	Dec 91	Born 6 lb 12 oz.
4 mths	Apr 92	Started going to childminder Kate.
5 mths	May 92	Learned to sit up.
6 mths	Jun 92	Held bottle with both hands.
8 mths	Aug 92	Spoke a few words like Mumma, Dadda, Baby.
10 mths	Oct 92	Started to bottom shuffle.
1 yr	Dec 92	Able to play with pop-up toys, open a book and turn pages, feed herself with finger food.
1 yr 3 mths	Mar 93	Able to stand up on her own.
1 yr 6 mths	Jun 93	Started losing interest in toys, rolling her

eyeballs back until they almost disappeared. Started to avoid eye contact.

1 yr 8 mths	Aug 93	Became frightened to go on swings and slides. Started biting her hands. Stopped using her hands except for holding the bottle.
1yr 9 mths	Sep 93	X-ray on Emma's legs.
1 yr 10 mths	Oct 93	Started walking independently.
1yr 11mths	Nov 93	Speech and language therapy assessment.
2 yr	Dec 93	Started crying incessantly, biting her hands and grinding her teeth. Psychological assessment. Portage assessment.
2 yr 1 mth	Jan 94	1st appointment with paediatrician, co-ordination test.
2 yr 1 mth	Jan 94	Left Kate's care. Started attending local nursery and pre-school assessment centre.
2 yr 2mths	Feb 94	Hearing test, sight test and blood test.
2 yr 3mths	Mar 94	Genetic tests – Down's Syndrome, Fragile X, Torch screen.

2 yr 4 mths	Apr 94	2nd appointment with paediatrician – to discuss results from tests between February and April.
2 yr 5 mths	May 94	High and low frequency hearing tests Neurological tests.
2 yr 7 mths	Jul 94	EEG (Electro-encephelogram) Brain Scan.
2 yr 8 mths	Aug 94	Hearing test, Eyesight test.
2 yr 9 mths	Sep 94	Tentative Diagnosis of Rett Syndrome.
2 yr 10mths	Oct 94	Confirmed diagnosis of Rett Syndrome.
3 yr 6 mths	Jun 95	Started BIBIC programme. Improvement in mobility.
4 yr 8mths	Sep 95	Started attending special unit in a mainstream school. Improvement in social skills.
5 yr 11mths	Nov 97	Started cranial acupuncture in China. Improvement in posture and feeding skills.
6 yr 8 mth	Sept 98	Started attending special school for children with severe learning difficulty. Improvement in self awareness.

9 yrs 1mth	Jan 01	Visited Australia, Hong Kong and Singapore.
10 yrs	Dec 01	Had a 10th birthday party.
13 yrs	Dec 04	Became a teenager.
14 yrs	Sept 05	Started having teenage tantrums.
15 yr 7 mth	Jun 07	Started wearing a moulded jacket to stop scoliosis getting worse.
18 yrs	Dec 09	Had an 18th birthday party.

Appendix C

Resources

WEBSITES
General carers
www.carers.org
Princess Royal Trust for carers

www.carersuk.org
Carers UK

www.caringwithconfidence.net
Caring with Confidence: Courses for carers

www.crossroads.org.uk
Respite Care

www.nhs.uk/carersdirect
NHS Carers Direct: Information and support for carers

www.vitalise.org.uk
Short term break for disabled people and their family

www.expertpatients.co.uk
Expert patients: Courses for patients and carers

Disability
www.cafamily.org.uk
Contact a Family

www.disabilitynow.org.uk
Disability Now

www.mencap.org.uk
For people with learning disability

www.nas.org.uk
National Autistic Society

Mental illness
www.anxietyuk.org.uk
For people who suffers from anxiety and phobias

www.mentalhealthcare.org.uk
Mental Health information for friends, families and carers

www.mind.org.uk
National Association for Mental Illness

www.moodgym.anu.edu.au
Mood gym – free Cognitive Behaviour Therapy

www.rethink.org.uk
About mental illness

www.time-to-change.org.uk
Campaign to end mental illness discrimination

Older People
www.firststopcareadvice.org.uk
One stop service for older people, their families, gives advice, information on housing, care, money and rights.

www.ageconcern.org.uk
Age Concern

www.alzheimers.org.uk
Alzheimer's Society

www.parkinsons.org.uk
Parkinsons Disease Society

Drug and Alcohol Addictions
www.alcoholics-anonymous.org.uk
Support for people with alcohol problems

www.addaction.org.uk
Drug and alcohol treatment charity

www.phoenix-futures.org.uk
Services for people with drug and alcohol problems

Bibliography

Argent, Hedi, *One of the family*, BAAF, Skyline House, 200 Union Street, London SE1 OLX, 2005. A handbook for kinship carers. Fostering children. The child care system etc, where to get help. Also stories of dysfunctional families.

Battison, Toni, *Caring for Someone with Depression*, Age Concern England.

Carers and Disabled Children – House of Commons Bills No. 13 – EN (Session 1999 – 2000), Stationery Office Books.

Douglas, Anthony and Terry Philpot, *Caring and Coping. A Guide to Social Services*, Routledge. The management and day-to-day work of the social services in Britain.

Golding, Rachel & Liz Goldsmith, *The Caring Person's Guide to Handling the Severely Multiply Handicapped*. All about movement, Good illustrations.

Greenman, Jan, *Life at the Edge. Living with ADHD and Aspergers Syndrome: The true story of Luke's life with labels*. Hullavington: J Greenman (self published).

Hancock, Ruth et al, The *Long Term Effects of Being a Carer* – Studies in Ageing, Stationery Office Books.

Henry, George, *The Carer*, Vanguard Press.

Heywood, Bernard, *Caring for Maria Alzheimer's*. Element Books.

Highe, Jackie, *Now Where Did I Put My Glasses? Caring for your parents*. Simon & Schuster, 2007.

Hogg, Gil, *Caring for Cathy*. Leicester: Matador. Fiction. About a traffic accident victim suffering from Huntingdon's chorea.

Howard, Helen, *Caring for someone in their own home*. A handbook for friends and family. Age Concern Books, Age Concern England, co-published with Carers UK. Contains useful addresses, and further reading on caring tasks related to depression, cancer, heart problems, diabetes, alcohol problems and dementia.

Irwin, Colin, *In Search of Alison*.

Johnstone, Matthew. *Living with a Black Dog*, Robinson Publishing, 2009. A personal account of depression.

Lee, Elizabeth, *In your own time*: *A guide for patients and their carers facing a last illness at home*. O.U.P. Oxford Medical Publications, 2002. Advice for the terminally ill.

Lewis Jackie and Debbie Wilson, *Pathways to Learning in Rett Syndrome*, David Fulton, 1998. Both teachers, Jackie a mother of a RS child. Foreword by Yvonne Milne, Founder and President of Rett Syndrome Association UK.

Lindberg, Barbro, *Understanding Rett Syndrome*, Cambridge, Mass: Hogrefe & Huber. 2nd edition, 2006. Foreword by Dr Andreas Rett, Vienna. Based on 80 Swedish girls interviewed in 1986. Details of physical problems and guidance on treatments.

Mace, Nancy L. & Peter V. Robins, *The 36-Hour Day*. Warner, 2006. Caring for an Alzheimer's sufferer within the family.

McCall, Bridget, *The Complete Carer's Guide*, Sheldon Press. Aimed at informal carers.

McDonald, Ann, *Understanding Community Care*: *A guide for Social Workers*. CacMillan, 1999.

Marriott, Hugh, *The Selfish Pig's Guide to Caring*, Piatkus, 2006.

Carers have to look after themselves as well. A personal account of how to deal with heavy burdens. These can include other people's unhelpfulness and feelings of guilt brought about by isolation and fatigue. Strategies that work are described, with humour. His wife had Huntingdon's disease.

Matthew, Jane. *The Carer's Handbook: Essential Information and Support for those in a Caring Role.* How To Books, 2007. Foreword by Judith Cameron, author of The Guardian's *Who Cares?* Columns. She has a daughter with Encephalitis lethargica, profound brain damage. Covers all the practical considerations.

Munitch, Brenda, *The Little Book of Positive Thoughts for Carers.* Youwriteon.com.

Picault, Jodi, *Handle with Care.* Hodder & Stoughton. Fiction. Charlotte's daughter Willow was born with a very severe form of brittle bone disease. When the family faces financial disaster Charlotte is advised that she could sue her doctor for wrongful birth.

Read, Jim, et al. *How To Cope as a Carer.* MIND.

Sillers, Stuart, *A Workbook for Carer Workers*, MacMillan, 1992.

Spink, Henrietta, *Henrietta's Dream.* Hodder, 2004. A personal story, not a how-to. A courageous mother with two profoundly disabled sons seeks doctors world wide. The Henry Spink Foundation Charity, established in 1996, helps parents with disabled children (see resources).

Sutcliffe, David, *Introducing Dementia: The essential facts and issues of care.* Age Concern England. Aimed at professionals, this is an introductory guide to caring for sufferers at home and in long-term carer situations.

Uncertain Futures: *People with Learning Difficulties and Their*

Ageing Carers. Pavilion Publishing (Brighton) Ltd.

Whitfield, Ann, *Make the Most of Being a Carer*. Need2Know, 1998. The author is a social worker with a disabled child. She runs support and pressure groups for carers of disabled children.

Young, Pat, *Welfare Services: A guide for Care Workers*. Macmillan, 1997.

Inspirational

M. Scott Peck, *The Road Less Travelled*. Arrow Books, 2006. First published 1978. The Ten Million Dollar Bestseller. Facing our difficulties and suffering through the changes, leading to self understanding.

Peiffer, Vera, *Positive Living*. Piatkus, 2001. Positive Thinking.

Persaud, Dr Raj, *Staying Sane. How to Make Your Mind Work for You*. Index Books. 2007. Bantam Books, 2001.

Pessin, Andrew. *The God Question*. What Famous Thinkers Have Said About The Divine. One World Publications, 2009.